Living
WITH
Anxiety

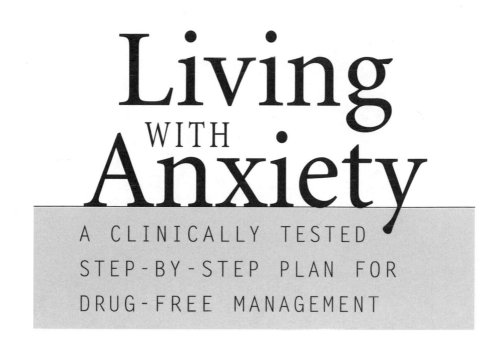

Living
WITH
Anxiety

A CLINICALLY TESTED
STEP-BY-STEP PLAN FOR
DRUG-FREE MANAGEMENT

Dr. Bob Montgomery
and
Dr. Laurel Morris

PERSEUS PUBLISHING
Cambridge, Massachusetts

Text design by Tonya Hahn.
Set in 12-point Minion by Perseus Publishing Services.

Cataloging-in-Publication data for this book is available from the Library of Congress.
ISBN 1-55561-306-3

Perseus Publishing is a member of the Perseus Books Group.
Find us on the World Wide Web at http://www.perseuspublishing.com

Perseus Publishing books are available at special discounts for bulk purchases in the United States by corporations, institutions, and other organizations. For more information, please contact the Special Markets Department at Perseus Books Group, 11 Cambridge Center, Cambridge, MA 02142, or call (800) 255-1514.

2 3 4 5 6 7 8 9 10—04 03 02

Contents

Introduction

This book is mainly for people having problems with anxiety or with an anxiety disorder, such as panic attacks, phobias, posttraumatic stress disorders and obsessive-compulsive problems. Reading the early chapters will help you decide whether you have a problem with anxiety and, if so, what kind of problem. Reading and working through the later chapters will help you tackle your anxiety problem effectively.

Psychologists, counselors and other mental-health professionals who work with people suffering from anxiety problems can use this book as an aid. It provides explanations of those problems, which can help the sufferer feel less dismayed by them, and it sets out step-by-step instructions drawn from current research and clinical practice. It is intended to provide mental-health professionals with a structured program they can adapt to each person's needs, thus facilitating cost-effective therapy or counseling and also helping maintain any gains the person makes in therapy.

This book deals only with anxiety-based problems. Your level of anxiety reflects the level of stress in your life. We will not consider in detail any major sources of stress that contribute to your anxiety, such as a bad job or a troubled marriage. However, we do describe post-traumatic stress disorders in chapter 8 and outline some steps for both preventing and managing them. But, if your anxiety problem is mostly the result of a current or recent crisis experience, we recommend you use our book *Surviving: Coping with a Life Crisis.*

SELF-HELP OR PROFESSIONAL HELP?

Self-help manuals have a mixed record of success. Some are helpful, some are not and some, particularly pop psychology books on sexual problems, can even make people worse. We have based this book carefully on current research and established clinical practice and we are confident that it will be helpful and not harmful.

However, successful self-help depends on three factors that are under your control:

1. You need to correctly identify your problem as one of anxiety rather than something else. The early chapters in this book should help you to do that with some confidence.
2. You need to be reasonably sure that you do not have some other significant problem that may be contributing to or complicating your anxiety problem. Again, the early chapters should help you to decide this.
3. You should follow our suggestions reasonably closely. We don't mean to be rigid and you can adapt our advice somewhat to suit yourself. However, sometimes people make what they think are small changes to a procedure that in fact make a big difference in how it works. If you have a lot of trouble applying one of our suggestions, it could mean that you have not correctly identified your problem, or that you have not recognized some interfering complication, or that you have not understood the instructions. Whichever of these applies, it may be time to think about getting some professional help.

> We have based this book carefully on current research and established clinical practice and we are confident that it will be helpful and not harmful.

The people who do best at self-help are usually those with relatively uncomplicated problems and reasonable self-confidence. They can see themselves being successful at a self-help project. We encourage you to try self-help because it can build your self-confidence to see yourself solving your problem on your own—and it's more cost-effective than consulting someone. But if you are not successful at self-help or if, after you have seen what it entails, you think it's too much for you, then we encourage you to seek professional help. This is not a sign of weakness. It's common sense.

> We encourage you to try self-help because it can build your self-confidence to see yourself solving your problem on your own—and it's more cost-effective than consulting someone.

We suggest you consult a qualified clinical psychologist. In the United States, look for a psychologist who is board certified by the American Board of Clinical Health Psychology, an affiliated board of the American Board of Professional Psychology. In Canada, look for a psychologist who is accredited by the Canadian Psychological Association or who has a postgraduate qualification in clinical psychology. Don't be afraid to ask. A responsible professional will not be offended and you might save yourself a lot of wasted effort and money.

Unfortunately, if you don't have health insurance, or if your insurance doesn't cover (or inadequately covers) mental health, seeing a psychologist can be expensive. If you cannot see a qualified clinical psychologist, then consult some other kind of counselor or therapist. Just remember this rule of thumb: If you don't feel like you're getting much help after a few consultations, with anybody, you probably won't get much help in the long run. We encourage you to exercise your rights as a consumer and find help somewhere else.

WHAT ABOUT MY DRUGS?

Because anxiety problems are common and because most medical practitioners have not learned any other way of helping, many people with anxiety problems are prescribed drugs. We consider the problems and risks of this approach in detail in chapter 3. We also give you a plan for weaning yourself off unnecessary drugs.

Even if you think the drug is not helping you, you should wait to wean yourself off until you work through chapter 3. If you have been taking the drug for any length of time, your body will have adapted to it. If you just stop taking it, you risk having a withdrawal reaction, which can be very unpleasant. You don't need an extra problem right now. So let's get to work on your anxiety problem.

1

What Is Anxiety?

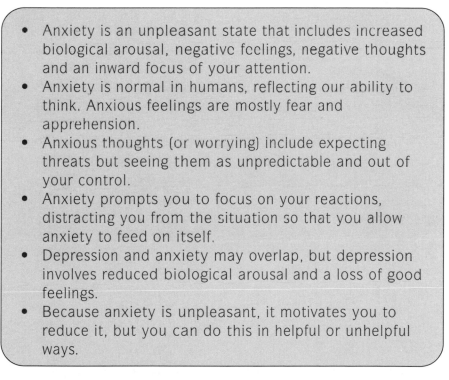

- Anxiety is an unpleasant state that includes increased biological arousal, negative feelings, negative thoughts and an inward focus of your attention.
- Anxiety is normal in humans, reflecting our ability to think. Anxious feelings are mostly fear and apprehension.
- Anxious thoughts (or worrying) include expecting threats but seeing them as unpredictable and out of your control.
- Anxiety prompts you to focus on your reactions, distracting you from the situation so that you allow anxiety to feed on itself.
- Depression and anxiety may overlap, but depression involves reduced biological arousal and a loss of good feelings.
- Because anxiety is unpleasant, it motivates you to reduce it, but you can do this in helpful or unhelpful ways.

You may be surprised to learn that psychologists have not finally agreed on what anxiety is. Given the number of people who suffer from excessive anxiety and its related problems, you might expect that we would know it inside out. Unfortunately, not yet. Because it is such a common problem, anxiety has sparked a great amount of research, which is still going on and generating a number of competing theories. Don't worry; if you are already having trouble with anxiety, you don't need an extra dose of confusion, and we won't give you one. We will not discuss the scientific debate over the nature of anxiety. If you are interested in that, you can read some of the books listed in our Further Reading section at the end of the book.

It can certainly be unpleasant, although mild levels of anxiety can heighten your level of excitement in pleasant ways. Notice how people line up to pay money for horror movies and roller coaster rides.

We will give you just one theory about anxiety, based mostly on the ideas of Dr. David Barlow, professor and director of clinical programs at the University of Vermont. We think he has done an excellent job of combining much of the latest research to give an up-to-date and sensible theory of anxiety.

We can give you an up-to-date idea of what anxiety is and how best to manage it. But, as with other fields of active scientific research, some of what we say will undoubtedly be revised in the future. In the meantime, you can be confident that we have given you the benefit of the latest research and our own and others' clinical experience.

A WORKING DEFINITION OF ANXIETY

Anxiety is an unpleasant state that includes

- negative emotions (for example, you feel fearful, nervous, jittery, distressed or upset)
- expecting unpleasant or threatening events, inside or outside yourself, but seeing them as unpredictable and out of your control

- shifts in your attention to focus needlessly on the possible threats and your reactions to them.

Before we describe these components in more detail, we want to emphasize that we regard anxiety as normal in humans. It can certainly be unpleasant, although mild levels of anxiety can heighten your level of excitement in pleasant ways. Notice how people line up to pay money for horror movies and roller coaster rides. In people with no sexual problems, some anxiety can actually increase their sexual arousal. Excessive anxiety can be or cause a problem, or we wouldn't be writing this book, but to experience some anxiety seems to be the natural lot of humans.

Anxiety in Different Cultures

Researchers have found that something like anxiety exists in most, if not all, other cultures and that the nature of the anxiety process tends to reflect the characteristics of each culture. For example, Chinese people may complain of a problem called *pa-leng*, an apparently exaggerated fear of losing body heat, which they believe results from an imbalance between the life forces, *yin* and *yang*. Iranians may complain of "heart distress," describing physical symptoms centering around the heart but bearing a strong resemblance to a Western panic attack. There are well-documented folk magic rituals in a number of cultures, such as voodoo dolls in the Caribbean and "pointing the bone" among Australian Aborigines, which seem to involve scaring the victim to death by causing an intolerably high level of anxiety.

Using standard checklists of anxiety symptoms, researchers have found similar levels of anxiety in different cultures. Which symptoms people complained of, how they explained the symptoms to themselves and, therefore, what was effective help for them varied from culture to culture. But anxiety itself seems to be a universal and therefore normal part of being human.

ANXIETY AND EMOTIONS

You will notice that anxiety is not simply an emotion; it is a state that includes a number of possible unpleasant emotions. Different people may report different feelings as a part of anxiety. You may feel differently in different anxiety-provoking situations. But the basic flavor of the emotions involved in anxiety is fear and apprehension.

The current theories agree that human emotions include more than just the emotional feeling itself but also the thoughts you have about the situation and your biological reactions, including activity in your nervous and hormonal systems. There is disagreement as to which comes first or what causes the other, but we won't concern ourselves with those questions. At this stage they won't make any difference in our practical suggestions for managing your anxiety.

Our working definition of anxiety includes a number of possible negative emotions. So it must also include the thoughts associated with those emotions, which we discuss shortly, and the biological reactions, which we won't detail in this book. The use of drugs to treat anxiety problems is an attempt to get at their biological basis and we intend to convince you that it is not usually a wise or successful attempt. You can learn to relax physically as a part of managing your anxiety successfully. You don't need a detailed understanding of the biological basis of emotions in order to relax.

ANXIETY AND THOUGHTS

Anxiety occurs in response to possible threats you can see coming. This is one of the aspects of anxiety that make it a peculiarly human reaction. Many animals will react with fear in the face of a threat, but humans can anticipate a threat before it happens, imagine one that isn't happening or remember one from the past. Some psychologists have said that it is our human ability to think, which serves us so well in many ways, that also makes us capable of anxiety and vulnerable to its problems.

ANXIETY AND FEAR

Fear is the natural reaction of animals, including humans, to an immediate threat. It is adaptive (or useful) if unpleasant because it activates us to do something to protect ourselves. Even that definition needs to be finely tuned: We need an amount of fear that matches the degree of threat, enough to get us making an appropriate response to deal with the threat. With too little fear we may react too little or too slowly and the threat may overtake us. Too much fear and we, like other animals, will probably freeze rather than react constructively.

If fear is the natural reaction to an immediate threat, what is anxiety? It is the natural reaction to a possible threat, rather than a present one. This is where your thoughts first come into anxiety. Anticipating coming threats, imagining possible threats and even remembering past threats can all trigger anxiety.

The thoughts associated with anxiety have two major themes:

1. You see the possible threats as unpredictable, even though you are expecting them. You may be unsure about when a threat will arrive, how strong it will be, exactly what form it will take or whether it will happen at all. You may be unsure about how you will react and how the situation will turn out, although with higher anxiety there tend to be more negative expectations: thoughts of not coping with the threat and of having the situation turn out badly. This uncertain and unclear expectation of something going wrong is the apprehensiveness that is central to anxiety.
2. The second theme in anxiety-related thoughts is the belief that you lack control over the situation. This can include believing that you will not be able to prevent, or effectively react to, the threat and that you will not be able to control

your own reactions. Our working definition of anxiety includes expectations of unpleasant events, both inside and outside yourself.

Part of your anxiety may be that you expect to handle the outside situation badly, to fail, perhaps to make a fool of yourself. The more problematic your anxiety, the more likely it is that some of your thoughts will be critical evaluations of yourself and your reactions. So, part of your anxiety may be the expectation of handling your inner reactions badly, perhaps losing control. Later we'll explain how these are important elements of the anxiety problem in panic attacks.

ANXIETY AND WORRY

Worry involves thinking about a possible problem, what you might do about it and how it might turn out. Like fear and anxiety, worrying is normal in humans and can be adaptive. Being able to anticipate a threat before it happens can give you time to think out what to do about it. Worrying that leads to constructive preparation and action can be smart. Anxiety is an arousing state, presumably in preparation for coping with the expected threat.

ANXIETY AND ATTENTION

The third part of our working definition of anxiety is a shift in and narrowing of your attention. As anxiety builds, your attention moves away from other things, including the problem, to focus narrowly on your bad feelings, your biological reactions or your thoughts about the unpredictability of the threat and your lack of control in the situation.

The nature of this attention focus can reflect the nature of your anxiety. For example, someone feeling anxious about possible sexual failure will focus his attention on anything that suggests he is about to fail, distracting himself from what is going right in his sexual activity. This focus contributes to the exact problem he fears. Someone feeling anxious about spiders tends to become oversensitive to anything that suggests spiders. Someone feeling anxious about having a panic attack will focus her attention on the internal signs of arousal, such as quicker breathing or heart beating, which may signal the beginning of a panic attack.

Especially, but not only, in the case of a panic attack, narrowing and focusing your attention can become a negative loop, feeding on itself. You can start to worry about feeling anxious, making yourself even more anxious. In this state, you may feel unable to shut off or control your anxiety.

ANXIETY VERSUS DEPRESSION

Some psychologists have argued that anxiety and depression overlap so much that there is little point in distinguishing between them. Certainly people's scores on anxiety and depression tests tend to correlate, to be similar to each other. But the two states do differ in some ways that are important, which suggests that the best approaches to managing them will also be different.

While both anxiety and depression involve unpleasant emotional feelings, the negative feelings of anxiety center on the presence of fear and apprehension while the negative feelings of depression tend to reflect an absence of positive feelings. Anxiety is associated with biological and psychological arousal, apparently in preparation for coping with the expected threat. Depression is associated with a biological slowing down and reduction in activity. While the thoughts in both states include ideas of helplessness, anxious thoughts focus on expected if unpredictable threats and your reactions to them and depressed thoughts focus on a more general sense of hopelessness about the future and lots of self-criticism and self-blame.

> While both anxiety and depression involve unpleasant emotional feelings, the negative feelings of anxiety center on the presence of fear and apprehension while the negative feelings of depression tend to reflect an absence of positive feelings.

Of course, it is possible for someone to be both anxious and depressed and for elements of these two states to overlap. For our purposes, we don't need to separate them completely, except to say that we do not deal directly with depression in this book.

ANXIETY AND MOTIVATION

Anxiety is an unpleasant state, as you have probably noticed or you wouldn't be reading this book. Because it is unpleasant, it can motivate you to end or at least reduce your anxiety. This again can be adaptive. Feeling anxious about a coming problem may prompt you to take some constructive steps to prepare for it. Your anxiety has served its useful purpose and goes away or at least lessens. On the other hand, humans have a remarkable ability to react to anxiety in self-defeating ways. These reactions may reduce your anxiety, but at other, higher costs, or they may reduce your anxiety only temporarily, to have it return with a vengeance. This is when your problems may begin.

2

Problems with Anxiety

Some anxiety is normal and can enhance your performance.

- Anxiety becomes a problem when it is intense or prolonged, when it prevents you from functioning normally or when it causes other problems.
- Anxiety differs from the Type A Behavior Pattern (TABP). Anxiety involves an inward self-focus; the TABP involves an outward focus on the task.
- Anxiety is triggered by stress, which is the process of coping with life demands. Some people seem to be more vulnerable to reacting to stress with excessive anxiety.
- Anxiety problems are so common that they probably constitute the single largest mental health problem.
- More women than men complain of anxiety problems, especially agoraphobia.
- Some people do not see anxiety problems as serious, but excessive anxiety is associated with high death rates, including by suicide.

Anxiety is normal and some anxiety can be helpful, arousing you to prepare yourself for a coming demand. Since 1908, psychologists have known that moderate amounts of anxiety enhance your performance, a fact so well established that it is now called the *Yerkes-Dobson Law,* after the two psychologists who first described it. It is often depicted in the graph as follows:

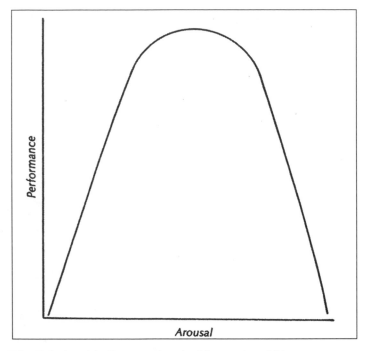

The Relationship Between Level of Arousal and Human Performance

At too low a level of arousal, you may put little or no effort into the task at hand. At medium levels of arousal, you are up and running, giving your best performance. As your arousal level increases further, your performance is disrupted and declines. This high level of arousal is unpleasant in itself and, by disrupting your performance, it can cause you additional negative consequences. This is where anxiety problems lie.

Anxiety becomes a problem when it

• is intense or prolonged
• prevents you from functioning normally and successfully

- triggers self-defeating behavior, such as panic attacks, phobias, obsessive-compulsive habits or drug dependence

Dr. Barlow (see page 2) proposes that what distinguishes normal, adaptive anxiety from problematic anxiety is the shift in your attention away from the relevant task. This shift causes your performance to decline. Focusing your attention on yourself—your bad feelings, your biological reactions, your apprehensive thoughts or your expectations of loss of control and failure—increases your anxiety. So your attention shifts even further and your performance declines even more.

ANXIETY VERSUS THE TYPE A BEHAVIOR PATTERN

Some psychologists say this focus on the self distinguishes people with anxiety problems from those with the Type A Behavior Pattern. A person with TABP is sometimes called a "workaholic" because people with it tend to lead unbalanced lifestyles, overinvolved in work to the detriment of their marriages, families and health. They may be materially successful, but they may also be easily divorced or dead. Their overinvolvement in work makes them unavailable to their marriages and families, causing inevitable problems. Although some medical experts are reluctant to accept the findings, we think there is good evidence to show that the TABP contributes to heart disease, because it is usually associated with high levels of anger. There is clear evidence linking the hormone changes produced by anger with changes in your blood cells that will contribute to heart and blood vessel disease.

In 1983, researchers reported that people with a TABP have a strong *external* focus of attention, unlike the inward shift of attention with anxiety. Because they have a strong need to feel in control, they tend to focus fully on the task in hand, even ignoring potentially serious physical symptoms. People with problems from a TABP tend to have the same physical symptoms as people with anxiety problems, but they don't report the same level of bad feelings or the same kind of negative thoughts. We think this is because they are more inclined to deny any bad feelings as signs of "weakness." Most think it's OK to be angry, however, because that prompts aggression, which is "strong."

The TABP as just as big a problem as excessive anxiety, with high risks to your important relationships and your health. We also think it actually *reduces* your real success rate in life, especially over any length of time. But it is not an anxiety problem and we will not deal with it any further in this book.

ANXIETY AND STRESS

Despite the popular attention given to stress in recent years, or maybe because of it, stress is frequently misunderstood. Much of what is suggested for stress-management is ill-informed, too simplistic or just plain fraudulent. We will not be considering stress at length in this book because it is such a big topic it rates a book of its own. But it is involved in anxiety, so we will give you a basic introduction.

Dr. Charles Spielberger is professor of psychology at the University of South Florida and generally regarded as a leading authority on stress. He defines stress as the interaction between your coping skills, on the one hand, and the demands of your life, on the other hand. Stress is the process of coping with your life. In this sense, stress is a normal part of being alive. In fact, moderate stress levels are good for you, resulting in your best performances, health and well-being, as in the Yerkes-Dobson Law mentioned above. It is immoderate levels of stress that cause stress-related problems.

> Stress is the process of coping with your life. In this sense, stress is a normal part of being alive.

Dr. Spielberger sees anxiety as the reaction to stress. He describes the stress process as beginning with a demand on you, which you see as a threat, causing you to react with anxiety. He draws a distinction between anxiety as a *state,* meaning how anxious you feel at any time, and anxiety as a *trait,* meaning how much you are prone to react to stress with anxiety. Different people have different degrees of this anxiety trait, making them more or less vulnerable to anxiety.

Dr. Barlow draws more of a distinction between stress and anxiety but comes up with a similar theory. He suggests that people with anxiety problems are more likely to have strong biological reactions to demands (or stress). He reviews some research that suggests this biological vulnerability may be inherited genetically. These biological reactions produce bad feelings, especially if you cannot explain them to yourself satisfactorily and react with the self-focused attention described above. People with anxiety problems are inclined to misinterpret all these reactions, particularly seeing things as out of control and unpredictable.

We won't concern ourselves with any theoretical differences among the experts. Both are saying that stress from your life can lead to anxiety and that some people are more vulnerable than others to reacting that way. The issue of stress tends to focus on the demands in your life and your ability to deal with them—your coping skills. The issue of anxiety tends to focus on your reactions to those demands and how you handle those reactions—your anxiety management skills. Although these two issues obviously overlap and interact, we will stick with that distinction, too.

If you think your problem reflects too many demands in your life and inadequate skills for coping with them—the problem is more *outside* you—you are probably facing a stress problem. If you think your problem reflects your reactions to life's demands and inadequate skills for managing those reactions—the problem is more *inside* you—you are probably facing an anxiety problem.

HOW ANXIOUS AM I?

Chances are, if you're reading this, you already believe you have too much anxiety. However, if you would like a more specific idea of how high your anxiety level is, you can take the test below. (This test has been developed by Dr. David Burns, who is director of the Behavioral Sciences Research Foundation at the Presbyterian Medical Center of Philadelphia.) Even if you don't need to have your anxiety problem confirmed for you, this test may be helpful in a different way. You can use it to record your progress in reducing your anxiety by taking it every week or two. In that case, don't write your answers on the test form. Instead, use the answer sheet (or a copy) that follows the test.

Your total score on the test can be interpreted according to the box of scores above. How did you do? Sometimes people doing tests like this in our clinic are upset when they get high scores. It can be disturbing to have to confront a problem and accept that you do have it and it is big. But accepting that you have a problem is the first, absolutely necessary step in tackling it. A high anxiety score may be bad news, or it may just confirm what you already expected. Either way, it is a clear starting point to measure your progress from.

The Burns Anxiety Inventory

Instructions: Following is a list of symptoms. Put a (✔) in the space to the right that best describes how much that symptom or problem has bothered you during the past week. If you would like a weekly record of your progress, record your answers on the separate answer sheet (see page 17) instead of filling in the spaces in the test itself.

SYMPTOM LIST CATEGORY 1: ANXIOUS FEELINGS	0-NOT AT ALL	1-SOMEWHAT	2-MODERATELY	3-A LOT
1. Anxiety, nervousness, worry or fear				
2. Feelings that things around you are strange, unreal or foggy				
3. Feeling detached from all or part of your body				
4. Sudden unexpected panic spells				
5. Apprehension or a sense of impending doom				
6. Feeling tense, stressed, uptight or on edge				

CATEGORY 2: ANXIOUS THOUGHTS	0-NOT AT ALL	1-SOMEWHAT	2-MODERATELY	3-A LOT
7. Difficulty concentrating				
8. Racing thoughts or your mind jumping from one thing to the next				
9. Frightening fantasies or daydreams				
10. Feeling that you're on the verge of losing control				
11. Fears of cracking up or going crazy				
12. Fears of fainting or passing out				
13. Feeling of physical illness or heart attacks or dying				
14. Concerns about looking foolish or inadequate in front of others				
15. Fears of being alone, isolated or abandoned				
16. Fears of criticism or disapproval				
17. Fears that something terrible is about to happen				

(continues)

SCORE LIST

Total Score	Degree of anxiety
0–4	Minimal or no anxiety
5–10	Borderline anxiety
11–20	Mild anxiety
21–30	Moderate anxiety
31–50	Severe anxiety
51–99	Extreme anxiety or panic

CATEGORY 3: PHYSICAL SYMPTOMS	0-NOT AT ALL	1-SOMEWHAT	2-MODERATELY	3-A LOT
18. Skipping or racing or pounding of the heart (sometimes called palpitations)				
19. Pain, pressure, or tightness in the chest				
20. Tingling or numbness in the toes or fingers				
21. Butterflies or discomfort in the stomach				
22. Constipation or diarrhea				
23. Restlessness or jumpiness				
24. Tight, tense muscles				
25. Sweating not brought on by heat				
26. A lump in the throat				
27. Trembling or shaking				
28. Rubbery or "jelly" legs				
29. Feeling dizzy, lightheaded or off balance				
30. Choking or smothering sensations or difficulty breathing				
31. Headaches or pains in the neck or back				
32. Hot flushes or cold chills				
33. Feeling tired, weak or easily exhausted				

Add up your total score for the 33 symptoms and record it here: _____

Date: _____

The Burns Anxiety Inventory Answer Sheet

Instructions: Put a 0, 1, 2 or 3 in the space to the right after each of the thirty-three symptoms from the previous pages, depending on how much it has bothered you in the past week: 0 = Not at all; 1 = Somewhat; 2 = Moderately; 3 = A lot. Then add up your total score for all 33 symptoms at the bottom.

1.	1.	1.	1.	1.	1.	1.
2.	2.	2.	2.	2.	2.	2.
3.	3.	3.	3.	3.	3.	3.
4.	4.	4.	4.	4.	4.	4.
5.	5.	5.	5.	5.	5.	5.
6.	6.	6.	6.	6.	6.	6.
7.	7.	7.	7.	7.	7.	7.
8.	8.	8.	8.	8.	8.	8.
9.	9.	9.	9.	9.	9.	9.
10.	10.	10.	10.	10.	10.	10.
11.	11.	11.	11.	11.	11.	11.
12.	12.	12.	12.	12.	12.	12.
13.	13.	13.	13.	13.	13.	13.
14.	14.	14.	14.	14.	14.	14.
15.	15.	15.	15.	15.	15.	15.
16.	16.	16.	16.	16.	16.	16.
17.	17.	17.	17.	17.	17.	17.
18.	18.	18.	18.	18.	18.	18.
19.	19.	19.	19.	19.	19.	19.
20.	20.	20.	20.	20.	20.	20.
21.	21.	21.	21.	21.	21.	21.
22.	22.	22.	22.	22.	22.	22.

(continues)

23.	23.	23.	23.	23.	23.	23.
24.	24.	24.	24.	24.	24.	24.
25.	25.	25.	25.	25.	25.	25.
26.	26.	26.	26.	26.	26.	26.
27.	27.	27.	27.	27.	27.	27.
28.	28.	28.	28.	28.	28.	28.
29.	29.	29.	29.	29.	29.	29.
30.	30.	30.	30.	30.	30.	30.
31.	31.	31.	31.	31.	31.	31.
32.	32.	32.	32.	32.	32.	32.
33.	33.	33.	33.	33.	33.	33.

Total Score
Today's Date

ANXIETY PROBLEMS
ARE COMMON

Anxiety problems are common. Researchers have found that 30 to 40 percent of the general population have sufficiently high levels of anxiety to benefit from professional help. A recent survey found the following:

- 4 percent of the U.S. population suffer from general anxiety problems
- about 1 percent, panic attacks
- about 3 to 6 percent, agoraphobia
- about 2 percent, social phobia
- about 5 to 10 percent, simple phobias
- about 2 percent, obsessive-compulsive problems

These percentages may not seem very high, until you apply them to the whole population. For example, they suggest that more than 10 million Americans suffer from general anxiety problems, and more than 8 million suffer from agoraphobia. Because many people with problems will go first to their medical doctor and medical doctors are usually poorly trained in psychology, not all anxiety problems are correctly identified, at least not at first. Many of the patients referred to heart specialists because of chest pain turn out to be suffering from panic attacks. Another study found that 36 percent of patients going to their medical doctor had had at least one panic attack in the previous year. Dr. Barlow concluded that these recent surveys showed anxiety problems to be the single largest mental health problem in the United States!

> Researchers have found that 30 to 40 percent of the general population have sufficiently high levels of anxiety to benefit from professional help.

ANXIETY AND WOMEN

Another disturbing fact that emerges from these surveys is that anxiety problems are apparently more common in women than men. This seems to be especially true of agoraphobia. In the United States, 75 percent of agoraphobics are women. We don't know why this is so. It may only be that it is more acceptable for women than men to say they suffer from anxiety and fear, or that men have learned to "tough it out" more. It may be that men are more willing to "treat" themselves for excessive anxiety, for example with excessive alcohol. It may be that the difference reflects hormonal differences between men and women, which may make women more vulnerable to anxiety. Or it may reflect cultural differences in the way men and women are raised, particularly in regard to the

> Many of the patients referred to heart specialists because of chest pain turn out to be suffering from panic attacks.

desirability of being "in control." It is interesting to note that the TABP, which involves a focus on staying in control of the situation, is more common in men than women.

Whatever the explanation turns out to be, women definitely complain of anxiety more often than men do. Along with the fact that anxiety problems are common, anyway, this seems to have had the unfortunate effect of making some people not take anxiety problems very seriously. Some people, ignorant about the real nature and effects of stress, are inclined to dismiss stress problems as unimportant, "all in the head," or as evidence of weakness or an attempt to shirk responsibilities. Similarly, anxiety problems are often regarded lightly. If the patient is a woman, her anxiety is likely to be dismissed with labels such as "suburban neurosis" or "housewife's syndrome."

> Some people, ignorant about the real nature and effects of stress, are inclined to dismiss stress problems as unimportant, "all in the head," or as evidence of weakness or an attempt to shirk responsibilities.

ANXIETY PROBLEMS ARE SERIOUS

Anxiety problems can be serious. Sufferers of anxiety problems, especially people with panic attacks, have higher death rates. These higher rates are due to higher rates of suicide and higher rates of heart and blood vessel disease in people with anxiety problems. Most people associate suicide with depression, not anxiety, and it is true that depression with strong feelings of hopelessness can lead people to suicide. But recent research suggests that anxiety is also associated with suicide, at least as much as depression is. We don't yet know whether this is a direct link or whether it reflects the fact that many anxiety sufferers will later develop depression or drinking problems, but it underscores the potential seriousness of anxiety problems themselves.

We are not discussing the potentially serious problems associated with excessive anxiety to add to your gloom, but rather to add to your motivation to tackle this program steadily. You may not need convincing, but there may be others in your life, including family and professional helpers, who would benefit from reading this and the next chapter. Anxiety is normal. Excessive anxiety is unpleasant and a potentially serious problem, in itself and because of the other problems it can cause. One of the most common problems is drug dependence. If you have been using a drug, whether prescribed, social or illegal, to manage your anxiety, there is a risk that continuing to use it will interfere with your success on our program. So, before we go on with anxiety management, we consider that possibility in the next chapter.

Practical Exercise

If you have not already done it, complete the Burns Anxiety Inventory on pages 14–16, both to measure your present anxiety level and to give you a starting point from which to measure your progress. Copy the answer sheet so that you can take the test again, every week or so.

3

Anxiety, Drugs and Drug Dependence

- Because anxiety is unpleasant, some people try to reduce it with drugs.
- There is a strong link between anxiety and dependence on drugs, both social (including alcohol) and illegal.
- Anxiety often triggers health-reducing behavior, such as bad eating and drinking habits and smoking.
- Because alcohol probably increases anxiety, tackle your drinking problems *now*.
- Drugs usually prescribed for anxiety problems may make them worse, often have bad side-effects, leave you vulnerable to anxiety again when you stop taking them and have a high risk of being addictive.
- Antianxiety drugs are prescribed at high rates for women and older people. In older people they can cause symptoms such as dementia and dangerous falls.
- To avoid bad side-effects, to get the most from this program and to avoid being addicted and the risk of

> withdrawal symptoms, we advise you now to
> gradually wean yourself off antianxiety drugs. This
> is most safely done with the help of your doctor.

Anxiety is an unpleasant state, so it motivates people to do something to reduce their anxiety. Sometimes that's helpful, because it prompts you to tackle your problems constructively.

Sometimes that's not helpful, because it may prompt you to use a drug to reduce your anxiety. Any drug you use to manage your anxiety is never going to be your best answer and can easily become a big problem itself. There is a large amount of research now linking anxiety with all forms of drug abuse.

ANXIETY AND DRUG ABUSE

Despite the impression you get from the media and the movies, our society's major drug problems are with legally available drugs, including alcohol. One study found that 33 percent of a group of 102 alcoholics had either agoraphobia or social phobia at a severe level, while another 35 percent had the same phobias at milder levels. Another study found 18 percent of a group of 60 alcoholics had severe agoraphobia or social phobia, while another 35 percent had the same phobias at milder levels. In both studies, more than half of the alcoholics had identifiable anxiety problems. In general, people with anxiety disorders are 1.7 times more likely to have a substance abuse problem.

Any drug you use to manage your anxiety is never going to be your best answer and can easily become a big problem itself.

These are typical of the studies showing a strong relationship between anxiety problems and drinking problems. This is an especially unfortunate link because recent research shows that alcohol does not actually reduce anxiety and may even worsen it. It now seems likely that some people start using alcohol to manage their anxiety and initially obtain some apparent relief. However, the recent research shows that, when alcohol is digested, one byproduct is a chemical that actually increases your anxiety level. The risk is that you then reach for another drink, to try to get your anxiety down again, and there you are with an alcohol-dependence problem.

Clinical research and experience in helping people quit smoking identify anxiety as a common trigger for smoking. Many smokers report that they feel they need to smoke in order to cope with daily tension and anxiety.

Accepting alcohol and tobacco as our major social drug problems is not intended to belittle the problems for those who become dependent on illegal drugs. They are numerically less, but they also have to contend with the high prices and doubtful purity and dosages of their illegal drugs and the clandestine world their drug dependence draws them into. More recently they face the additional risk of contracting AIDS if they share needles. Although small in number, users of illegal drugs represent a major cost to the whole community, through both the loss of their productivity and the crime many of them resort to in order to pay for their drugs, as well as the organized crime that sucks its blood money from them.

We will not consider drug abuse in detail in this book. For at least twenty years psychologists have been pointing out that effective help for people with drug abuse problems needs to include effective help in anxiety management. People more experienced in the drug field than we are have concluded that the "drug war"—trying to reduce drug abuse with a tough legal approach—has failed. This is evidenced by the rising rates of drug abuse and related crime. We can see possible advantages in the controlled supply of drugs to users, but we hope it will be accompanied by the availability of anxiety management and other relevant help.

ANXIETY AND HEALTH

In chapter 1 we report the alarming fact that anxiety problems are associated with high death rates. Some of this is due to the unexpectedly high rate of suicide associated with anxiety problems.

If you have been seriously thinking that suicide might be the answer to your problems, we suggest you now work through chapter 15 and consider having a discussion with a qualified clinical psychologist or other counselor. In chapter 15, we share with you some evidence that suggests that suicide is rarely the best answer to anyone's problems, including anxiety.

There is plenty of research and clinical experience showing that anxiety is a common trigger for health-reducing behavior.

But not all of the higher death rate associated with anxiety problems is due to suicide. Some of it is due to physical illness, particularly heart and blood vessel disease. These are diseases that largely reflect your lifestyle, what and how much you eat and drink, whether you smoke, and whether you exercise. There is plenty of research and clinical experience showing that anxiety is a common trigger for health-reducing behavior. Many people eat or drink unwisely or smoke tobacco because they feel anxious. A binge or a drink or cigarette offers some temporary relief.

We explained in detail earlier just how temporary and self-defeating the relief from drinking is. There are similar drawbacks to using food or tobacco for anxiety reduction. The two eating problems, anorexia (starving yourself) and bulimia (vomiting after binge eating), both have strong anxiety components. The nicotine in tobacco may give you an immediate calm down, but only until the dose wears off. The health-damaging effects of smoking tobacco, on you and the people around you, are beyond reasonable question.

Overdosing on caffeine will increase your arousal level and therefore your vulnerability to anxiety (and poor sleep). Many people improve their mood (and their sleep) by using caffeine more sensibly.

If anxiety has prompted you to develop some health-reducing behavior, such as smoking, excessive drinking or bad eating habits, including anorexia or bulimia, we suggest you work on anxiety management using this book. At the same time, we suggest you start to work on your health-reducing behavior.

We realize this may seem like a tall order. You may understandably think you have enough on your plate just trying to do an anxiety management program. OK, if your health-reducing behavior involves eating or smoking, it won't hurt much to postpone tackling that until you are well on your way through this program. But, if your health-reducing behavior has been excessive drinking, you should start to do something about that now. As we explained above, alcohol has a high risk of increasing your anxiety, especially if you drink a lot of it. This is just going to undermine your progress on your anxiety management program. Consider any number of support groups or see a qualified clinical psychologist or other counselor.

Practical Exercise

Think about and write down your answers to these questions: Has anxiety caused you to develop any bad eating habits? Drinking habits? Smoking habits? If so, when do you plan to tackle them? How? Remember, it is best to tackle any bad drinking habits now, rather than later. Too much for self-help? Where will you go for some professional help?

_____

_____

_____

_____

_____

_____

ANXIETY AND PRESCRIPTION DRUGS

The link between anxiety and problems with social and illegal drugs is sad enough. Even sadder is the fact that, for many people, their anxiety-related drug problem is with drugs that have been prescribed for them, supposedly to help with their anxiety. This is a truly staggering problem, because of its size, because of its severity, because it results from good but misguided intentions and because it is going on today.

In 1994 a total of 18 million prescriptions were given for antianxiety drugs and 25 million prescriptions for antidepressants (a number of which are also used to treat anxiety). These numbers have been on the rise ever since. Between 1995 and 1999, drug expenditures in the United States increased from $65 billion to $125 billion (yes, billion!). From the above figures we know that a large share of this was spent on antianxiety drugs. If all this expenditure was genuinely helpful to anxiety sufferers, we might see it as justified. But the truth is, antianxiety drugs are often used in unhelpful and even dangerous ways.

HOW CAN A DRUG HELP?

If excessive anxiety results from stress in your life interacting with a biological vulnerability, a tendency to focus on yourself, negative thinking habits and a lack of confidence in your ability to cope, how are these factors changed by taking an antianxiety drug? Obviously the only factor modified by the drug is your biological reaction. That may provide relief from your excessive anxiety, but obviously only for as long as you take the drug. The drug does not change the stress in your life, improve your coping skills, alter your habit of self-focus, make your thinking habits any less negative nor improve your self-confidence.

As many people have discovered, when you stop taking the drug, you are just as vulnerable to excessive anxiety as before. A growing number of research studies show that many people, sometimes most, whose anxiety problems were improved by taking an antianxiety drug relapse back into anxiety after stopping the drug. Researchers testing a new antianxiety drug on people with panic attacks found nearly a 100 percent relapse rate when the drug was stopped, with the patients having worse panic attacks than before.

> The drug does not change the stress in your life, improve your coping skills, alter your habit of self-focus, make your thinking habits any less negative nor improve your self-confidence.

This analysis would suggest that there may be a useful role for antianxiety drugs in helping people cope with a critical level of anxiety, to get them through a rough patch. In fact, we think there may be a reasonable argument for such a brief therapeutic use of antianxiety drugs in some cases. But the limited drug treatment should be accompanied by effective training in anxiety management, to reduce your vulnerability to excessive anxiety in the future, and a determination to stop using the drug as soon as possible. Unfortunately, this is not how most antianxiety drugs are used.

PRESCRIBED-DRUG DEPENDENCE

Boston psychiatrist and Harvard Medical School faculty member Dr. Joseph Glenmullen points out that many patients take SSRIs (such as Prozac, Paxil, Zoloft, Luvox and Celexa) for years at a time. Other studies ranging over 8 months to 6 years indicate that around 50 to 78 percent of patients taking antipanic medication continue the medication following acute treatment trials. This high rate of long-term use of antianxiety drugs reflects two factors.

First, most people feeling bad will initially go to their medical doctor. Most doctors are poorly trained in diagnosing and treating psychological problems, just as psychologists are not trained in medical problems. Certainly most doctors would sincerely like to help their troubled patients. Doctors are bombarded with advertising by drug companies, claiming that antianxiety drugs are effective and safe. Ashley Wazana, M.D., of McGill University, analyzed 29 studies of relations between doctors and the pharmaceutical industry and found that pharmaceutical companies spend $8,000 to $13,000 per year on each doctor for gifts, free meals, travel, educational programs and product samples. This, of course, doesn't include the $1.1 billion dollars in direct-to-consumer television advertising pharmaceutical companies spent in 1999 alone. Under these circumstances, it is not surprising that some doctors continue to prescribe antianxiety drugs in large and continuing amounts.

The second factor behind high rates of long-term use is that, despite the drug companies' claims to the contrary, antianxiety drugs have a high risk of being addictive. According to John Steinberg, medical director of the chemical dependency program at Greater Baltimore Medical Center, the United States produces 1.5 million Xanax addicts each year. Studies now indicate that 35 to 78 percent of patients who abruptly stop certain antidepressants (including tricyclic antidepressants and SSRIs, both commonly prescribed for anxiety disorders), after several months of treatment, will develop one or more withdrawal symptoms.

Some medical administrators and doctors have questioned whether the high rate of long-term antianxiety-drug use represents drug dependence or even a problem. Many people who have used these drugs for long enough to become dependent and then tried to stop taking them would not share their doubts. The withdrawal symptoms they have had to cope with have been severe enough to convince these poor patients of the undesirability of long-term use. We are convinced. People with anxiety problems do not need the additional burden of a drug-dependence problem.

> To make matters worse, antianxiety drugs are disproportionately prescribed for two groups: women and the elderly.

To make matters worse, antianxiety drugs are disproportionately prescribed for two groups: women and the elderly. We have already commented on the sexist tendency of some doctors to trivialize women's complaints and too quickly prescribe a drug, rather than investigate the complaint carefully or consider an alternative treatment, such as referral to a specialist. We suspect the poor treatment of the elderly in this regard reflects similarly stereotyped attitudes about old people, with disastrous results.

DRUGS AND OLDER PEOPLE

Adults age 65 and older take more prescription and over-the-counter medications than any other age group. In 1983, 25 percent of older adults used psychotherapeutic drugs regularly for sleeping problems, chronic pain and anxiety. In fact, 20 percent of older adults used a tranquilizer on a daily basis! This is particularly worrisome because other research has identified these drugs as a major cause of falls and fractures in the elderly.

A 1999 study of homebound elderly found that nearly 40 percent were prescribed at least one inappropriate drug, and 10.4 percent were prescribed two or more. High rates of inappropriate prescribing were found for such drugs as benzodiazepines, the most common antianxiety drugs, (41.3 percent) and antidepressants (27 percent). In addition, elderly people have a higher risk of adverse drug interactions because they are more likely to have multiple health problems that require multiple prescriptions.

In part, this is the responsibility of the older patient herself. Some will "shop around" among doctors, collecting a number of prescriptions, and wind up taking a cocktail of drugs. Some will use drugs they have obtained without a doctor's prescription. But this situation also reflects a lack of diligence on the part of some doctors who are too quick to reach for the prescription pad, especially when faced with an older woman whose complaints fall outside the doctor's expertise. It also reflects the marketing activities of the drug companies and the potency of some drugs that can be obtained without prescription. There is room here for some effective action by the medical and pharmaceutical professions and health authorities.

This tragic overuse and misuse of drugs by the elderly, with its serious and sometimes fatal side effects, also results from the effects of the drugs themselves. As many people who have tried antianxiety drugs can testify, to achieve a satisfactory reduction in anxiety, some users wind up in a zombie-like state. It's not surprising that some lose track of their drug-taking and accidentally overdose. The side-effects of many antianxiety drugs include the symptoms of dementia, such as memory loss, confusion and restlessness. In other words, many of the problems in older people that are blamed on their age are due to the drugs that may have been prescribed to "treat" those very problems.

SOUR GRAPES?

We are aware that some people may want to dismiss our concerns about the use of antianxiety drugs as reflecting the fact that, as psychologists, we are not trained in the use of and cannot prescribe drugs. We will make two points in reply. First, we do know a fair amount about and are not simply opposed to the use of drugs. Dr. Montgomery's doctoral research involved using drugs (from the antidepressant group) to study the nerve circuits in the brain involved in motivation. He has published more than twenty research papers in international journals of psychopharmacology and related fields, the ones that report drug research. Dr. Morris's honors research involved the combined use of a drug and psychological treatment to help women with stubborn sexual problems. We have helped a drug company prepare a combined drug and psychological program for managing weight in people having trouble controlling their appetite. We are not simply antidrug. We are strongly opposed to the unnecessary, unhelpful and unhealthy use of drugs, which is clearly occurring with most antianxiety drugs.

Second, our concerns are shared by many *medical* authorities. In 1991, Samuel Cohen, professor of psychiatry (not psychology) at the London Hospital Medical College, said that he has found many phobias are *caused* by antianxiety drugs and alcohol. He reported that 45 percent of his patients with anxiety problems were taking antianxiety drugs or alcohol and that, if they stopped using the drug or alcohol, they recovered from their anxiety problems. He also expressed concern over the effects of these drugs in the elderly and concluded that drugs should never be used to treat anxiety. There are nondrug alternatives.

That's what this book is all about. We have deliberately titled it *Living with Anxiety,* not *Eliminating Anxiety,* because that's not our goal and it shouldn't be yours. By strengthening your anxiety-management skills, you should be able to live successfully with anxiety, as humans normally do. If that means you occasionally feel bad when anxiety is high, we think that's a better quality of life overall than what is offered to you by antianxiety drugs. We hope you are about to prove this to yourself.

NEW DEVELOPMENTS IN DRUG THERAPY

There is always a lot of research being done into drug therapies, and you may want to check out the latest news to help you decide whether or not to try some drug therapy for your anxiety problem. For example, as we report in detail in chapter 5, a new drug therapy and well-established psychological therapy have been shown to have the same effects on brain functioning in people suffering from panic problems. This gives us two effective ways of treating these problems, and some people will benefit more from one than the other, or from a combination of the two.

That's what this book is all about. We have deliberately titled it *Living with Anxiety*, not *Eliminating Anxiety*, because that's not our goal and it shouldn't be yours.

We suggest you seek this advice from someone who is up to date with the latest research and who has your interests at heart, rather than someone who has a bias in favor of either drugs or psychotherapy. This should be your family doctor or clinical psychologist, but unfortunately that won't always be the case. Don't be afraid to ask for a good explanation of whatever recommendations you are given, and don't accept a brush off. It's your problem, and it will eventually be your solution.

If you do find some drug therapy helpful, perhaps to help you out of an immediate hole as we describe in chapter 5 for people with panic problems, we still suggest that you aim eventually to cope without the drugs. You don't need a drug dependence problem instead of or, worse, as well as your anxiety problem.

TIME TO QUIT

If you have been using antianxiety drugs, our best advice is that you should consider stopping this now, for the following good reasons. First, the drugs have a high risk of actually being the cause of some of the symptoms you are blaming on your anxiety, as well as of other undesirable side-effects, as you have probably noticed for yourself.

Second, there is a risk that, if you learn new anxiety-management skills while you are taking a drug, you will not remember them well when you stop taking the drug. Psychologists have found that learning can be *state-dependent*, meaning that you remember it best only if you're in the same state you were in when you first learned it. On the other hand, you remember it badly in a different state.

Third, there is the risk that, if you have been using the drug for long, especially if you have become dependent on it, you may have unpleasant withdrawal symptoms when you do eventually stop. These symptoms may be so unpleasant that they cause you to relapse and set you back in your progress in anxiety management.

The fourth risk is an important one. Drug dependence has a strong psychological component, even when the user is also physically dependent on the drug. Believing that he needs the drug, that he can't cope without it, that he will feel horrible without it all contribute to a victim's drug-dependence. You may already have thoughts like these about your antianxiety drug, contributing to your continuing use of it. If you continue to use your medication while you work on this program, you risk seeing the improvements that result from this

> If you continue to use your medication while you work on this program, you risk seeing the improvements that result from this program as due to your drug.

program as due to your drug. That will only convince you all the more of your "need" to continue using the drug. You don't need to believe that fairy tale. It's time to quit.

WEANING YOURSELF OFF YOUR ANTIANXIETY DRUG

We completely accept that this is easier for us to suggest than it is going to be for you to do. You will probably feel anxious about your ability to cope without your antianxiety drug. If you have been taking the drug for long, you may suffer some unpleasant withdrawal symptoms. About 1 in 3 people cutting out their antianxiety drugs have some withdrawal symptoms, such as anxious trembling, dizziness, sweating, sensitivity to light or sounds, sleeping problems or nausea. You can minimize this risk by following the plan below for gradual reduction, with the assistance of your doctor. If you prefer to try the plan without your doctor's assistance, we encourage you to see a doctor if you have any strong physical symptoms or think that you might fail. We wrote this book because we believe in self-help, but we all need some outside help sometimes. In any case, you should *never* stop taking antianxiety drugs suddenly, especially if you have been taking many or if you have been taking them for a long time. There is a real risk of serious withdrawal symptoms, such as epileptic fits.

We suggest you share this part of your anxiety-management program with your doctor and get her or his help with it. To help you with this, we have written a letter to your doctor (below) to explain the plan for weaning you off antianxiety drugs. We suggest you ask your doctor to read the letter, as well as any other part of the book he or she wants. Then ask for help in doing the program. If your doctor won't help you wean yourself off antianxiety drugs, we suggest you ask why. If you are not satisfied with the explanation, ask another doctor.

Dear Doctor,

Your patient has started the self-help anxiety-management program detailed in this book. For the reasons we outline earlier in this chapter, we have advised your patient to wean him- or herself off antianxiety drugs now. If you would like to know more about those reasons, may we suggest you read this chapter? It won't take long.

Because of the need to adjust dose levels carefully and the possibility of some withdrawal symptoms, we have suggested your patient ask for your assistance in carrying out this gradual drug-reduction plan. Here's the plan:

1. Be aware that some patients, particularly those regularly using high doses of benzodiazepines, but even some using lower doses, need inpatient treatment and support while reducing their medication.

2. Establish the average daily dose for your patient. Your own medical records may be the most reliable guide to this, assuming you are the sole prescriber to this patient.

3. Reduce the dose in steps of 10 to 20 percent each week. A proportionate reduction like this seems to be more acceptable to patients than reducing by fixed amounts (e.g., 5 mg). We suggest that it is important to discuss and agree on each reduction with your patient. If problems occur during the reductions, consider switching to diazepam. Some patients tolerate diazepam better and find it easier to reduce dose levels using this.

4. Write your patient clear instructions for each week's dose level. Anxious people can be forgetful or confused.

5. Reassure your patient regarding the safety of a gradual withdrawal plan, but be prepared for genuine physical problems. Not all symptoms will be due to withdrawal.

6. Encourage your patient to seek alternative methods for managing anxiety by

A. working on this program, or other self-help material
B. consulting a qualified clinical psychologist or other good counselor
C. relaxation training, such as audiocassettes, yoga classes and relaxation groups

7. It will help if you can be available by phone, especially during the first two weeks. It usually takes only a few moments to reassure an anxious person, or you can encourage him or her to make an appointment with you or his or her counselor.

8. If somatic symptoms appear, you can reduce the dose more slowly. Consider using propanolol or clonidine, at appropriate dose levels.

9. If your patient appears to fail at the withdrawal program:

   A. Does he or she need referral, for face-to-face anxiety management, to a qualified clinical psychologist or other appropriate counselor?

   B. Is he or she obtaining prescriptions somewhere else?

10. It will help if you reassure your patient that you will continue to see him or her, for help with anxiety or sleeping problems, even when the medication has been stopped. As you will know, it is important that your patient knows that he or she can see you without the excuse of needing medication.

Thank you for taking the time to read this letter. We personally know how busy private and professional practice can be. We hope you will find it (and the rest of this book) helpful to you in helping your patients with anxiety problems.

Dr. Bob Montgomery and Dr. Laurel Morris

Practical Exercise

Have you been using antianxiety drugs? When will you make an appointment with your doctor to ask for his or her assistance in weaning yourself off? Be sure to take along our letter to share with your doctor. If you prefer to try for yourself, strive for the same 10 to 20 percent reduction in your dose level each week. But, if you develop any serious physical symptoms, do see a doctor.

— 4 —

General Anxiety

- A general anxiety problem involves feeling anxious most of the time, for at least six months, because of excessive worrying about at least two major life areas.
- This general worrying distinguishes general anxiety from other anxiety problems. It also shows itself in a number of physical symptoms and in being overalert.
- Antianxiety drugs are not helpful, certainly in the long run, not only because of the risks associated with their use but because they give small anxiety relief that lasts for only a short time.
- To manage a general anxiety problem, you need to change negative thinking habits, to learn to relax and stop worrying about feeling anxious, and to stop worry behaviors.
- If you have developed avoidance habits, it will help to tackle those, too.

General anxiety is sometimes called *free-floating anxiety* because it tends to permeate most of your life, rather than being focused on a particular part of it as are some anxiety problems, such as phobias or panic attacks. If you have general anxiety, you tend to feel anxious and tense all day, regardless of what situation you're in or what you're doing. General anxiety problems often begin between age twenty and forty and are equally common in men and women.

DO YOU HAVE A GENERAL ANXIETY PROBLEM?

Psychologists use a standard set of rules to decide what problem a person has. These rules are compiled in the *Diagnostic and Statistical Manual, Fourth Edition* (1994), and are meant to help in research (which won't concern you right now) and treatment (which will). The idea is that correctly identifying your problem allows you to select the most appropriate treatment. We will now describe the key points in those rules to help you decide if your anxiety problem is general anxiety.

The central feature of general anxiety is unrealistic and excessive anxiety because of lots of worrying. People with this problem often describe themselves as "chronic worriers." To be a general anxiety problem, your worrying should be about at least two major life areas. For example, one researcher found that people with general anxiety worried about similar common areas: family, then money, then work and then possible illness. Of course, you might also worry about some other life area. In fact, people with general anxiety tend to pick up on current issues in their lives and worry excessively about those, until something else comes along to worry about.

> People with general anxiety tend to pick up on current issues in their lives and worry excessively about those, until something else comes along to worry about.

This is different from the worrying that occurs in other anxiety problems, which tends to focus more narrowly and be more anticipatory. For example, someone with a panic problem will mostly worry about future panic attacks. Someone with a social phobia will worry mostly about future social situations in which she expects to fail. Someone with an obsessive-compulsive problem may worry mostly about germs or other contamination. You might worry about these sorts of things, too, but only as a part of more general worrying, if you have a general anxiety problem.

This excessive worrying needs to have been happening for some time, usually more than six months, to distinguish it from the quite normal distress reaction anyone might have because of a disturbing life event. If your current anxiety is probably a reaction to some recent crisis—being a victim of a crime or accident, coping with grief, being in a large-scale disaster, or any big upheaval in your life—then your problem is more likely to be a crisis reaction. In that case, you will find another of our books more helpful. We wrote *Surviving: Coping with a Life Crisis* for people coping with a life crisis of any kind.

People with general anxiety problems usually show a number of physical symptoms as well, such as

- trembling
- twitching
- feeling shaky
- muscle tension (which may cause aches or soreness)
- restlessness
- fatigue

They usually show signs of increased biological arousal, such as

- feeling short of breath, as if being smothered
- heart palpitations
- sweating
- clammy hands
- dry mouth
- dizziness
- feeling light-headed
- nausea
- diarrhea
- hot flashes

- chills
- frequent urination
- trouble swallowing or a "lump in the throat"

General anxiety often includes being overly alert, such as feeling worked up or on edge, being easily startled, having difficulty concentrating, disturbed sleep and irritability. To be sure you have a general anxiety problem, rule out the possibility that your anxiety symptoms are due to a physical problem. For example, problems with your thyroid gland or drinking too much caffeine can cause many of these symptoms. If you think that your symptoms may be physically caused, you should ask your doctor for a check-up.

People with general anxiety problems also may develop worry behaviors. These are behaviors that are meant to correct or prevent what you worry about. For example, you may frequently phone your spouse or children to make sure they're OK, or frequently check yourself for symptoms of a possible illness. Making checks like these is, of course, sometimes appropriate, but if you have a general anxiety problem, you will be doing them excessively. In fact, some people perform their worry behaviors so much that they become like rituals that the person feels compelled to go through. You may notice the similarity between worry behaviors and the compulsive behaviors we describe in chapter 9. People with obsessive-compulsive problems use their compulsive behaviors to reduce the anxiety caused by their obsessive thoughts. Likewise, some people with general anxiety problems use their worry behaviors to reduce the anxiety caused by their excessive worrying. The problem in both cases is that the anxiety reduction is only temporary, and meanwhile the person is

> To be sure you have a general anxiety problem, rule out the possibility that your anxiety symptoms are due to a physical problem. For example, problems with your thyroid gland or drinking too much caffeine can cause many of these symptoms.

spending a lot of time and energy on behavior that is really part of the problem rather than a solution. There are better ways of dealing with worrying thoughts (see chapter 11), and below we have some suggestions for dealing with worry behaviors.

How much does the above description fit your anxiety problem? Don't make this question something extra to worry about. You don't need to be absolutely certain which anxiety problem you have. In any case, they can overlap. For example, it's not unusual for someone with a general anxiety problem to have occasional panic attacks, but to worry about them less than someone with a panic problem. The practical point is that, if you think your problem fits the above description reasonably well, you should be following our plan below. If you decide that you also have some other problems with anxiety and you need to take other steps to tackle them, that won't hurt at all.

DO DRUGS HELP?

The drugs usually prescribed for general anxiety problems are the benzodiazepines, the antianxiety drugs we review in detail in chapter 3. Using these drugs for anxiety can cause major problems. These include the risk of side-effects that are as much of a problem as, and sometimes confused with, the original anxiety; the risk of physical addiction, making you vulnerable to serious withdrawal symptoms; and the risk of psychological dependence, undermining your self-confidence and making you vulnerable to relapsing back into anxiety when you stop taking the drug.

Dr. Barlow and his colleagues reviewed a lot of research evaluating these drugs and concluded that they offer only a small reduction in anxiety that lasts for only a few weeks. These findings reinforce our suggestion that, if benzodiazepines are used at all to treat general anxiety, it should only be for a short time during a particularly difficult period. The drug treatment should be stopped as soon as possible, to minimize the serious risks listed above, and should be accompanied by anxiety-management training.

There have been attempts to use other drugs, including some of the antidepressant drugs, to treat general anxiety. Overall these have not been very successful, although some (such as buspirone) do

seem to reduce anxiety without some of the physical risks associated
with benzodiazepines. We are frankly sceptical. The drug industry
has a long history of launching new drugs that are supposed to work
better than and have none of the risks of older drugs, only to have to
admit later that the new drugs also have their problems. Heroin was
developed as a "nonaddictive" replacement for opium. Amphetamines
were developed as "nonaddictive and completely safe" drugs for
reducing your appetite.

Even if antianxiety drugs that do not have the negative physical
side-effects of the benzodiazepines are developed, their use will still
leave people at risk of becoming psychologically dependent and of
relapsing back into anxiety when they stop taking them. We do not
see lifelong pill-popping as the answer to the problem of living with
anxiety.

MANAGING GENERAL ANXIETY PROBLEMS

Because the central feature of general anxiety problems is excessive
worrying, the main focus of managing them will be on changing
some of your thinking habits, as we discuss in chapter 11. Dr.
Barlow's group has been researching the effectiveness of different
kinds of treatments for general anxiety and has concluded that
helping people to change their negative thinking is the most
important. As part of this, we will tell you below how to tackle
worry behaviors.

Learning to relax also seems to help. We cover effective
relaxation techniques in chapter 12. To break your expectation of
being out of control and to stop your anxiety from feeding on itself,
you should work through chapter 10. These three chapters—10, 11
and 12—will be the backbone of a self-help plan for managing
general anxiety problems. You can add other units, if you think they
will be helpful. For example, if your anxiety problem has led you to
avoid social or sexual situations, work through chapter 13. If your
anxiety problem involves difficulty in dealing with other people,
work through chapter 14. *But work through chapters 10, 11 and 12
first.*

CONFRONTING YOUR WORRIES AND STOPPING WORRY BEHAVIORS

Because worry behaviors are being used much like the compulsive behaviors described in chapter 9, to counter anxiety created by your own thoughts, you can use much the same strategy to eliminate them. This involves confronting your worries and preventing your worry behaviors. The basic procedure for confronting unreasonable fears like your excessive worries is spelled out in detail in chapter 6, so you should read that too, but here's the basic plan.

1. Write a list of your main, current worries, the things you presently worry about most.

2. Arrange them in order of how anxiety-provoking they are for you. You are going to start by confronting the least worrying and work your way up.

3. Can you already imagine situations as though they were real? Paint yourself a good, vivid mental picture? If you can, skip to the next step. If not, practice this skill by imagining good, pleasant situations. Imagine what you would see, then what you would hear, then what you would smell or taste, any feelings of touch or movement, and how you would feel emotionally. Take your time to paint the picture in detail, finally focusing on your feelings in that imagined situation. Take as long as you need to become a good imaginer.

4. Now, take the worry at the bottom of your list—the least anxiety-provoking one—and imagine it happening. You should try to hold this image in your mind for at least thirty minutes, making it as vivid as possible and imaging the worst possible outcome. Follow the suggestion in chapter 6 of confronting anxiety until you feel 70 percent of your maximum possible distress. Then you are allowed to take a break, but *it is very important that you return to the exercise and keep working through your list of worries like this.*

5. Once you have vividly imagined the worst possible outcome for this worry, make yourself imagine some alternative outcomes. If you have trouble doing this, use the steps in chapter 11 to help you plan some constructive steps you could take about this worry or to realize that it almost certainly won't turn out as

badly as you have been imagining. It can give you encouraging feedback to record your progress in these exercise: what you worried about, how vividly you could imagine it, what alternative, constructive outcomes you could begin to imagine, and how anxious it made you feel. With persistent practice, you should steadily find your worries become less anxiety-provoking for you.

6. Now make a list of your common worry behaviors, those habits you have gotten into to try to deal with your worries. A good guide can be other people's reactions. For example, does your family complain that you do too much checking by phone? Keep a record of your worry behaviors so that you have clearly identified them and the worries that prompt them.

7. When you are confronting your worries, following the steps above, or experiencing your worries at other times, it is important that you now refrain from your worry behaviors. Yes, this will make you feel anxious at first; use the skills in chapters 10, 11 and 12 to cope with that anxiety. In particular, the coping statement from chapter 10 can help:

> I expect to feel anxious when I confront my worries and prevent myself from doing my worry behaviors, but I'll cope; I won't try to deny my understandable anxiety nor to avoid my worries, but I also won't only think about how badly they might turn out, because other outcomes are also possible; if this worry is something I can tackle constructively, I'll do that now rather than just worrying about it; if there's nothing I can really do about this worry, at least now, then I'll find something else to do that will occupy my mind pleasantly or constructively. I'm not obligated to make myself anxious with unnecessary worrying.

8. Do you need help to stop your worry behaviors? In chapters 6 and 9, we outline how to recruit valuable assistance for this kind of confrontation program and how to motivate yourself to stick to what can be a difficult but ultimately successful plan.

Practical Exercise

Carefully read the description of a general anxiety problem. Do you think this describes you? If it does, your anxiety management plan is to skip to chapters 10, 11 and 12 and begin working through them. Are you unsure? Review the following list of symptoms and check off those that apply to you on a regular basis.

Do you have symptoms not listed below? Perhaps you are experiencing a different form of anxiety, in addition to generalized anxiety. For example, many who suffer from general anxiety also have occasional panic attacks. If you suspect that you have more than one anxiety problem, finish working through chapters 10, 11 and 12 and then go back to read up on the other forms of anxiety.

If you have been using antianxiety drugs to manage your general anxiety problem, we strongly suggest you work through chapter 3 before any other chapter.

Common Symptoms of Generalized Anxiety

_ anxious and tense all day, regardless of situation
_ unrealistic and excessive worrying ("chronic worrying") that has been going on for more than six months
_ worrying that centers around at least two major life areas (such as family, money, work)
_ feeling on edge, overly alert
_ easily startled

_ difficulty concentrating
_ disturbed sleep
_ irritability
_ trembling
_ twitching
_ feeling shaky
_ muscle tension (which may cause aches or soreness)
_ restlessness
_ fatigue
_ feeling short of breath, as if being smothered

(continues)

_ heart palpitations

_ sweating

_ clammy hands

_ dry mouth

_ dizziness

_ feeling light-headed

_ nausea

_ diarrhea

_ hot flashes

_ chills

_ frequent urination

_ trouble swallowing or a "lump in the throat"

5

Panic and Agoraphobia

- Panic is a sudden attack of intense fear, including physical symptoms.
- People with panic problems have strong biological alarm reactions and they focus on them.
- Problems build when a person panics over false or learned alarms.
- Escape is a natural reaction to intense fear, so panic problems often involve situations in which escape is difficult. Agoraphobia is now seen as a fear of going into such situations or into situations in which help would not be available if panic occurred. It is really a fear of panicking away from support.
- Many agoraphobics depend on "safety signals" to get by.
- Some physical problems can mimic panic.
- Antianxiety drugs are not helpful for panic problems, but some newer antidepressant drugs can be!
- Treating panic problems and agoraphobia centers on confronting your fears, aided by several coping skills and, preferably, some support.

We will describe both panic problems and agoraphobia in this unit because, as you will see, they are closely related. Recent research suggests that somewhere between 3 and 6 percent of the population suffer from agoraphobia, while another 1 percent suffer from panic problems. Once again, these percentages may seem small until you apply them to the whole population—they add up to a lot of suffering. This is illustrated by the uncertainty about just how common agoraphobia is. We can't be sure because many agoraphobics find it too difficult to leave home, even for treatment, so they remain hidden from researchers.

Agoraphobia seems to be about three times more common in women than men; that is, 75 percent of agoraphobics are women. We say "seems" because there are now good reasons to doubt this apparent difference. Panic problems, as distinct from agoraphobia, are about equally common in men and women. As we are about to explain, agoraphobia is really a special kind of panic problem marked by avoidance of going out. If panic is as common in men as in women, why would agoraphobia be different?

The answer seems to be that men are more likely to manage their agoraphobia with alcohol. Researchers have found that many people with panic problems or agoraphobia try to manage their anxiety with alcohol and most of these drinkers are men. We have previously mentioned the strong link between anxiety problems and drinking problems. A second factor that probably contributes to the apparent difference is that it is more culturally acceptable for women to stay at home.

Panic problems and agoraphobia usually start in early adult life. Most people report these problems as starting in their twenties. This is later in life than for other phobias (see chapter 6), which suggests that these are really different kinds of anxiety problems. "Agoraphobia" is probably the wrong name for this problem, as we explain below (see page 56).

PANIC PROBLEMS

The word "panic" actually comes from the name of the Greek god Pan. If this name conjures up the flutelike tones of the pan pipes, you may be dismayed to learn that Pan, the god, is supposed to have enjoyed himself by suddenly jumping out of bushes and scaring people to death. From this myth came the word "panic," an adaptation that may be appropriate, because one of the common fears during a panic attack is that you are going to die, perhaps of a heart attack. This is very unlikely, however much you may believe it at the time. As we intend to convince you, panic attacks are an unpleasant inconvenience but not a threat to your life or your sanity.

Pan, the god, is supposed to have enjoyed himself by suddenly jumping out of bushes and scaring people to death. From this myth came the word "panic," an adaptation that may be appropriate, because one of the common fears during a panic attack is that you are going to die, perhaps of a heart attack.

Psychologists using the guidelines from the *Diagnostic and Statistical Manual, Fourth Edition*, define *panic* as the sudden onset of intense fear, apprehension or terror, often associated with feelings of impending doom. The panic will usually peak within ten minutes, often sooner. A full panic attack will also involve at least four of the following symptoms:

- shortness of breath or smothering sensations
- choking
- heart palpitations or faster heart rate
- chest pain or discomfort
- sweating
- faintness
- dizziness, lightheadedness or feeling unsteady
- nausea or upset tummy
- feelings of not being yourself or of unreality
- numbness or tingling sensations
- hot flashes or chills

- trembling or shaking
- fear of dying
- fear of going crazy or of losing control

Different people report different combinations of these symptoms and you may experience slightly different mixes on different occasions. Most people with panic problems report the heart palpitations, dizziness, fears of going crazy or losing control, sweating and shortness of breath. Most people with panic problems report many more than four symptoms. Some people will report panic attacks with less than four of the above symptoms. These are called minor attacks and are experienced as less intense than a full attack.

FEAR, ANXIETY AND PANIC

Dr. Barlow (see page 2) and his colleagues insist that panic is a unique experience and not just a high level of general anxiety. Several lines of evidence support this. Panic problems and general anxiety problems respond differently to drug treatment and to psychological treatment. This suggests that they are different in nature, but it is not firm evidence. More convincing is the fact that panic attacks tend to run in families and in identical twins, while general anxiety problems do not. This suggests that panic attacks involve an inherited vulnerability.

Don't misunderstand this point. Previously we have said that it is likely that all anxiety problems have some inherited basis, most likely a tendency to overreact biologically to threats. This is not peculiar to panic problems, just apparently more marked. The other important fact is that research in this area shows that environmental influences, including your past experiences, are more important than genetic influences. So don't be pessimistic if there is a history of panic problems in your family. You just need to give yourself some constructive and helpful experiences now. That's what this book is for.

Dr. Barlow's theory is that panic is actually fear. As we've said, fear is natural and useful because it warns you of an immediate threat and arouses you to deal with the threat. This is your normal alarm reaction. Sometimes we can be frightened unnecessarily, scared when it turns out that there was no real threat. In this case, your reaction is a false alarm. The fact that it was a false alarm does not make your fear any less real or unpleasant. In fact, it can make it worse because you see it as inappropriate or unexplained.

As we've mentioned, our human capacity to think seems to make us vulnerable to anxiety problems. This seems to be true of panic problems, too. If you walk near a wild animal to photograph it, you may scare it. It reacts with fear and trots away a little. You stand still and it no longer feels threatened. It calms down and you get a great photo. It doesn't get worked up over a false alarm.

But humans sometimes do, especially if the trigger for the false alarm isn't apparent. If you can't give yourself an acceptable explanation for your sudden increase in arousal, you may react by feeling anxious about it. The reasons you imagine for your increased arousal can add to your anxiety.

Another feature of humans complicates this situation: We are excellent learners. If you have a real or false alarm reaction, especially one that you can't explain to yourself, you can easily learn to associate your panic with what you can see (or sense in some way): for example, being in a particular place. This becomes a learned alarm, just as effective at making you frightened as a real or false alarm.

The anxiety you then feel about your apparently unnecessary and inappropriate alarm reaction involves the usual shift in your attention to focus on yourself, especially the physical signs of your arousal. It involves misinterpreting those physical signs, for example, as a heart attack. It involves seeing yourself as not being in control because your reaction makes no sense anyway. And it leads to those two common fears: of losing control of your behavior and of going crazy. This theory basically says that panic is an intense fear reaction to a false or learned alarm, which then triggers intense anxiety.

> The fact that it was a false alarm does not make your fear any less real or unpleasant. In fact, it can make it worse because you see it as inappropriate or unexplained.

People who develop panic problems seem to have strong biological arousal reactions to alarms and are inclined to focus on those reactions. This explains why those inner signs of biological arousal can also become learned alarms. Many people with panic problems can bring on a panic attack just by breathing quickly. Fast, shallow breathing was a part of their original panic experience and is now seen as a sign that they are about to have another panic attack. Another person might focus on increases in heart rate and panic about those.

There is growing evidence that apparently "spontaneous" panic attacks are in fact triggered by normal biological reactions to things such as mild exercise, sex, sudden temperature changes or increases in stress. One woman who consulted us about her panic problems had attacks that were triggered by the caffeine in a cup of coffee. Even panic attacks that occur while you are asleep may be triggered by biological events associated with sleep, such as the big muscle twitches that can occur in deep sleep or interruptions to your breathing (a problem called *apnea*).

PANIC AND CLAUSTROPHOBIA

In the end, people with panic problems are basically anxious about having another panic attack. They may say, for example, that their panic attacks are caused by going into airplanes or elevators or riding in cars, but these are really the situations that have become false or learned alarms for them. Although it is theoretically possible for any external situation (or any inner biological response) to become a learned alarm, you will notice there is one common feature to the examples we just listed. They all involve being confined: inside an airplane, an elevator or a car.

Fear is natural and can be useful. It can trigger life-preserving behavior of two basic kinds, to fight the threat or to escape from it. If the threat is likely to overwhelm you, it makes sense to escape. Our theory says that panic is intense fear, so it will naturally trigger a strong urge to escape. If you see that your ability to escape is blocked, that will inevitably increase your alarm reaction. Since a major part of panic problems is the fear of having another panic attack, this applies to both your ability to escape from the alarming situation or to escape from your alarming reaction to it.

Claustrophobia is usually defined as a strong fear of being confined, of being in a small space from which your escape is difficult or impossible. In the past, it has been regarded as another phobia, like those we will discuss in chapter 6. However, it now seems likely that some people apparently suffering from claustrophobia are really having a panic attack problem, in which they focus on their inability to escape from the situation that is triggering their panic attack or from the panic attack they expect to occur in that situation.

A pointer to this possibility would be whether your discomfort at being in confined places had an obvious learning history. For example, if you had a frightening experience in a car and your discomfort at being in cars clearly dates from then, you are probably suffering from a phobia. You don't have to have directly experienced the scare. You may have seen it happen to someone else (even in a movie) or heard about it. The point is that, directly or indirectly, you have probably learned your fear of being confined. In that case, you will benefit from working through chapter 6.

On the other hand, if there is no apparent history of your learning to fear being confined, you are probably experiencing this quite common part of a panic problem and you will benefit from our plan below.

PANIC MAY NOT BE A PROBLEM

There is plenty of evidence that occasional panic attacks occur relatively frequently among the general population. One recent study found that one-third of a group of presumably normal young adults had had one or more panic attacks in the previous year. These people, who had panic attacks but had not sought help for them, showed several characteristics:

- They were more likely to also have other anxiety problems or depression.
- They were likely to have less severe panic attacks.

- They were more likely to have had their panic attacks in response to an apparent alarm, such as public speaking, conflict with others, periods of high stress or taking exams.

Being able to explain your panic attack to yourself may both keep it milder and lessen the risk of it becoming a repeating problem. We will draw on these possibilities later.

AGORAPHOBIA

Agoraphobia has usually meant a strong and unreasonable fear (like other phobias) of going into open spaces, of leaving your home (strictly of going into the *agora,* which is Greek for "marketplace"). In the light of current thinking we should now redefine it as a fear of being in a situation in which you might not have help if you were to have a panic attack with its frightening or embarrassing symptoms.

This view of agoraphobia is supported by the fact that many agoraphobics will develop their own "safety signals": a place, person or thing they use to allow them to go out without too much discomfort. A "safety" person is someone that the agoraphobic believes will provide help in the event of a panic attack, so it is usually someone who knows about the problem. Most often this is the agoraphobic's spouse but sometimes it is another family member or a friend. Likewise a "safety" place is somewhere that the agoraphobic believes would offer support in the event of a panic attack. The most common "safety" object is a bottle of antianxiety pills, sometimes even one that is unused or empty! Dr. Barlow's group found that three-quarters of their agoraphobic patients used some sort of safety signal, and about a quarter used two safety signals.

A person's reliance on safety signals underscores the fact that his fear centers on the possibility of another panic attack, rather than simply on being in open places. Open places represent a lack of support if you have a panic attack, particularly if you are alone. "Alone" means not accompanied by someone who understands your problem. Many agoraphobics feel threatened by crowded places, such as shopping centers and supermarkets. Because agoraphobia actually represents an excessive fear of panic attacks, Dr. Barlow suggests a better term: *panphobia.*

Although safety signals may have helped you to be more mobile than you would have been without them, using them is another form of psychological dependence, just like the dependence some people develop for drugs or alcohol. If you continue to use a safety signal, you risk seeing any improvement you make as dependent on the signal instead of recognizing that you can depend on yourself. This adds the risk that suddenly losing your safety signal might scare you enough to provoke a panic attack. So a part of our plan will be for you to wean yourself off any safety signals you have been using.

The psychologists' guidelines *(Diagnostic and Statistical Manual, Fourth Edition)* say that you have agoraphobia if you have a fear of being in places from which escape might be difficult or embarrassing, or in which you think that help might not be available in the event of a panic attack or some other severe symptoms. If you don't actually fear a panic attack, the symptoms you fear might be dizziness or falling, not feeling yourself, feeling unreal, losing control of your bladder or bowels, vomiting or heart distress. As a result of your fears, you restrict your travel away from home, unless you can use a safety signal, or you feel very anxious when away from home.

You will notice that these symptoms feared by agoraphobics who apparently don't have panic attacks are like a panic attack, if only a limited one. For this reason, we are inclined to stick to the theory that agoraphobia is usually a special case of panic attack problems, in which the person has learned to avoid the situations in which she fears having a panic attack, at least without available support. In fact, it seems that most people with a panic problem develop at least some tendency to avoid "risky" situations.

Some researchers say they do find people in the community with agoraphobia but no panic problems. Yet clinical psychologists say that they rarely, if ever, see agoraphobia in a person who doesn't have panic attacks as well. Of course, it is possible for someone to develop a fear of going away from home for reasons other than fearing a panic attack. But, since these people apparently don't seek help from psychologists much, we don't know much about them or their reasons for restricting their movements. If you think you have agoraphobia, as the *Diagnostic and Statistical Manual* defines it, but no panic attacks, not even limited ones, see if you can pinpoint what it is you fear about going out. If you can identify it, then parts of this book might still be helpful to you. But if you can't, maybe it's time you saw a qualified clinical psychologist.

PHYSICAL CAUSES OF PANIC

A number of physical problems can cause symptoms like panic. Naturally, if one of these is your real problem, you should be seeking medical help for it. However, having one of these physical problems diagnosed by your doctor does not mean it is impossible for you to also have a panic problem. The physical problem may interact with a panic problem, triggering or worsening panic attacks.

Given this possibility, we suggest you first see your medical doctor, if you think you might have one of these physical problems or even if you aren't sure that you don't. If you do have a physical problem, follow your doctor's advice in treating it. If you are still troubled by panic attacks once that treatment is well under way, then you should go ahead with our program. Here are the possible physical problems:

Low blood sugar levels (hypoglycemia) can cause sweating, palpitations, weakness, dizziness, faintness and trembling. Although hypoglycemia has become a trendy complaint lately, it is actually uncommon and rarely associated with panic problems. Many of the people who consult us believing they have hypoglycemia turn out to have stress or anxiety problems. This illness can be clearly diagnosed by your medical doctor and often managed by sensible eating.

Thyroid gland problems can cause over- or under-doses of some hormones, which in turn can cause restlessness, shortness of breath, palpitations, increased heart rate, trembling or sweating, and occasionally panic attacks.

Cushing syndrome is the result of high levels of a hormone called *cortisol,* sometimes occurring after prolonged high stress. It usually causes depression but sometimes anxiety and panic.

Adrenal gland problems, particularly a tumor, can increase levels of hormones such as adrenaline. Because these are the hormones usually released during stress or anxiety, this physical problem closely mimics panic problems.

Epilepsy in a part of the brain called the temporal lobe is associated with a number of emotional disorders, including anxiety. It can cause symptoms such as sweating, palpitations and feeling unreal.

Excessive caffeine can cause panic symptoms, as we have mentioned earlier. In fact, many people with panic problems work them out for themselves and avoid drinking caffeine, but some don't realize how much they are giving themselves a problem. A safe and healthy level of caffeine is up to 300 milligrams per day. This is about three cups of brewed coffee, or about five cups of instant coffee, or about six cups of tea, or about seven glasses of cola a day. People vary in their sensitivity to caffeine (like other drugs) and how you brew your drink makes a difference in how much caffeine it has in it. So use these figures as a guideline only.

The *Diagnostic and Statistical Manual* now includes a problem called *caffeinism,* recognizing the large number of people in our society who are addicted to caffeine. In addition to contributing to anxiety and panic problems, excessive caffeine can cause other daytime problems, such as difficulty concentrating and disturbed sleep at night.

Middle ear problems can cause dizziness and unsteadiness, and consequently a fear of falling. One research group recently found that a number of patients with panic problems or agoraphobia also had some middle ear abnormalities.

Heart problems, especially a condition called *mitral valve prolapse (MVP),* were thought to be closely associated with panic problems. Extreme MVP can cause chest pain, palpitations, headaches and giddiness. However, more recent research using better diagnostic procedures now suggests that there is no link between MVP and panic problems. Of course, if you think you might have a heart problem, you should consult your medical doctor, if you haven't already.

The same advice applies if you think you might have any of the physical problems above. If anxiety, panic or agoraphobia have been a serious problem for you, you have probably already been to your doctor. If not, a checkup to screen for possible physical problems is a good idea.

DO DRUGS HELP?

We won't repeat our strong reservations about the use of the usual antianxiety drugs, the benzodiazepines, in anything but short-term emergency situations. If you are using or thinking of using these drugs to manage panic problems or agoraphobia, we suggest you now read chapter 3, if you haven't already. Some researchers have been trying an antidepressant drug called imipramine (Imiprin, Tofranil) to treat panic problems, but the results are still not clear. Imipramine does not seem to have any direct effect on panic attacks but it may increase the improvements gained from psychological treatment. One psychologist has suggested that it does this by reducing depression in some panic patients, while Dr. Barlow believes it reduces anxiety by reducing the amount of apprehension you feel.

Before you rush off to your doctor for a prescription, we should advise you that many people using these antidepressant drugs suffer such strong negative side effects that they stop taking them. Of those who continue with the drugs, many will relapse when they stop using them.

Current research using a strong benzodiazepine, aprazolam (Xanax), has claimed success in reducing panic attacks. Studies show that it also has high relapse rates (45 to 90 percent), rebound effects and withdrawal symptoms. Clinical trials of benzodiazepines and antidepressants showed that 30 to 75 percent of patients continued to experience panic attacks and follow-up studies show that 50 to 80 percent continue to have anxiety problems after discontinuing these drugs.

Some more promising results have been obtained using some of the newer antidepression drugs, called SSRIs (or, if you're interested in the technicalities, specific serotonin reuptake inhibitors, which just describes how they are thought to work in your nervous system). In a very interesting piece of research, using a technique that shows how different parts of the brain are working, it was shown that panic sufferers receiving drug therapy with an SSRI had the same changes in brain functioning as did panic sufferers receiving psychotherapy along the lines described below. This is very exciting news because it shows that both appropriate drug and psychotherapy are having the same biological effects; in that regard, neither treatment approach had an advantage over the other. This means we have access to two different treatment approaches, and you can try the one best suited to you.

Because panic problems can result in major restrictions on your lifestyle—the agoraphobia part of the problem—and you may have tried unsuccessfully for some time to cope with the problem, you as a long-term panic sufferer may become very distressed or depressed, even suicidal (see chapter 15), and have difficulty beginning the psychological program we outline below. If you are in that situation, you can consider asking your medical doctor to give you some immediate relief by prescribing an SSRI.

This is the sensible, short-term approach to drug therapy for anxiety problems that we introduced in chapter 3. We are not recommending you take SSRIs for the rest of your life, and we are not recommending that you do nothing else about your panic problem. We are recommending that, if your panic problem has you in such a mess that you can't think straight (an important part of our program), you gain some temporary relief with a drug therapy that research has shown to be helpful. As soon as you are feeling well enough, we strongly recommend that you work through the program below and wean yourself off the drugs (see chapter 3). This combined drug and psychotherapy plan will help you to get yourself out of your present hole, then to solve your panic problem in a way that means you are unlikely to relapse after you stop using the drug. That makes sense to us, and we hope it does to you.

MANAGING PANIC
PROBLEMS AND AGORAPHOBIA

There is now strong evidence that the most effective way to deal with unreasonable fears is to confront them. This is certainly true for the fear of having another panic attack, involved in panic problems, and the fear of being away from somewhere safe, involved in agoraphobia. The most important part of solving these problems will be confronting those fears. Since this is also the key to solving simple phobias, we have explained how to confront fears in chapter 6, which deals with simple phobias as well.

You will feel more confident in your ability to confront your fears if you have some coping skills up your sleeve. So your complete program includes learning how to manage your anxious feelings (work through chapter 10), how to manage your anxious thoughts about panic (work through chapter 11), and how to manage the physical signs of anxiety that threaten another panic attack (work through chapter 12). The active support of someone important, such as your spouse or some other close relative or friend, will help you persist at confronting your fears and not let yourself be scared off. If you and this helper cannot already communicate helpfully about your feelings, you and he should work through chapter 14 together.

Practical Exercise

Carefully read the descriptions of panic problems and agoraphobia and then fill in the checklist below. Are you reasonably sure you do not have one of the physical problems that mimics panic? Should you get a medical checkup? If you decide you do have a panic problem or agoraphobia, start to work through chapters 10, 11, 12 and then 6. If you've been using antianxiety drugs to manage your problem, we strongly suggest you now work through chapter 3.

Rule Out These Medical Problems First
If you have . . .
   sweating
   palpitations
   weakness
   dizziness
   faintness
   trembling
get checked for low blood sugar (hypoglycemia).

If you have . . .
restlessness
shortness of breath
palpitations
increased heart rate
trembling or sweating
occasional panic attacks
get your thyroid gland and adrenal gland checked out.

If you have . . .
depression
some anxiety and panic
get checked for Cushing syndrome.

If you have . . .
sweating
palpitations
feelings of unreality
get checked for epilepsy.

If you have . . .
all the symptoms of an anxiety and panic problem, but especially
difficulty concentrating
disturbed sleep at night
you may have a caffeine problem (see page 59 for daily caffeine guidelines).

If you have . . .
dizziness and unsteadiness
a fear of falling
get checked for middle ear problems.

If you have . . .
chest pain
palpitations
headaches
giddiness
get checked for heart problems, particularly for mitral valve prolapse.

6

Phobias

- A phobia is an intense fear of something, accompanied by anxiety about confronting it, which causes you to avoid it to a degree that interferes with your life.
- You probably learn a phobia, directly or indirectly, and it is possible to develop a phobia of anything.
- Because people avoid their phobias, they unintentionally keep the phobia going.
- To overcome a phobia, you confront your unreasonable fears gradually, with the assistance of some coping skills and possibly a helper. This is also the way to tackle the fear of panic involved in panic problems and agoraphobia.
- Antianxiety drugs are not helpful with phobias.
- A motivational contract can help you stick to confronting your fears.
- Overcoming a blood phobia requires an extra technique.

A *phobia* is an intense fear of an object or situation, usually accompanied by anxiety about the possibility of confronting the object or situation, so that you tend to avoid it. As a result, the fear is interfering with your life in a significant way. What sets a simple phobia apart from other anxiety problems is its specificity, that you feel the intense fear only in response to your particular phobic object or situation. This makes it different from, for example, a general anxiety problem.

But we also distinguish between intense fears and phobias. Remember, fear is normal and can be useful. Feeling fear, even intense fear, of snakes, for example, can be understandable and may prompt you to avoid genuinely risky situations. That's not a problem and your fear is not a phobia. In fact, psychologists have found that snakes were the most common object of intense fears in the general population, followed by heights, flying, being enclosed, illness, death, injury, storms, going to the dentist, traveling alone and being alone. Intense fears are not unusual and not necessarily a problem.

On the other hand, if your fear of snakes is so extreme that you will not go into your backyard, where there is little real risk of meeting a snake, and this is interfering with your life, you have a phobia. This usually also means that you feel anxious about and avoid going into places where you think there might be snakes. The same psychologists found that the most common simple phobias were, in order of frequency, of illness or injury, storms, animals, death and heights.

> It is possible for someone to develop a phobia of just about anything, given the necessary circumstances.

These are common phobias, but it is possible for someone to develop a phobia of just about anything, given the necessary circumstances. "Discovering" new phobias has become a popular sport among some psychologists, more recently taken up by some journalists and Hollywood scriptwriters. It isn't hard. Just find the Greek name for something and tack on "phobia." For example, *acarophobia* is fear of insects, *agyiophobia* is a fear of crossing the street, while *aichmophobia* is a fear of sharp, pointed objects. And we aren't even out of the A's yet!

This kind of labeling for the sake of labeling is a waste of time as far as we are concerned, so we won't pursue it. You can decide you have a simple phobia if your problem involves intense fear of a specific object or situation, usually accompanied by anxiety about confronting that object or situation, and interference with your ability to lead a normal life. But take some time to ask yourself whether you don't have a more general problem with anxiety (see chapter 4) or other problems complicating your phobia, such as high stress (see the Introduction). If you can't decide, or your self-help work on your simple phobia isn't successful, consider seeing a clinical psychologist or other counselor.

SIMPLE PHOBIAS

Simple phobias do seem to be different from other phobias. They usually begin during childhood, although not always. For example, animal phobias on average start at around seven years old, blood phobias at around nine and dental phobias at around twelve. In contrast, agoraphobia and claustrophobia (see chapter 5) and social phobias (see chapter 7) all usually start later in life. Simple phobias seem to be twice as common among women as men, although this might again reflect different degrees of willingness to report being frightened, or men's use of alcohol for self-medication.

Clinical psychologists don't see many people complaining of just a simple phobia. Often people who see a psychologist about simple phobias also have other anxiety problems, high stress or another psychological problem. Yet we know from surveys that phobias are reasonably common, affecting from 5 to 10 percent of the population. It seems that many people with just a simple phobia decide to put up with it, rather than get any professional help. Although this will mean some interference with their lives if it meets our definition of a phobia, it is interference that they choose to cope with.

WHAT CAUSES A PHOBIA?

You may be pleased to learn that simple phobias are fairly easy to
treat successfully. Because we don't see many uncomplicated phobias
and because they are fairly easy to treat, they have not been as
thoroughly studied as some other anxiety problems. This shows in
the fact that we are not yet sure how you get a phobia, although
some sort of learning is the most likely explanation. At present,
psychologists believe that there are three ways in which you might
learn a phobia.

The first, most obvious way is by having a direct frightening
experience with the object or situation. After all, if you were savagely
attacked by a dog, it would not be surprising if you wound up
frightened of dogs. One psychologist found that 30 percent of his
patients with driving phobias had had an actual frightening
experience in a car, such as a collision. Another researcher found
that 68 percent of people with dental phobia had had previous
painful experiences at the dentist. But you will notice these figures
mean that many people with phobias have had no actual direct
contact with their feared object or situation. They have learned their
phobias indirectly.

Second, you can learn a phobia by watching (or hearing or
reading about) someone else having a frightening experience. The
more you identify with that person, the more you will be able to
imagine that her experience might happen to you. Two other factors
influence this way of learning a phobia: 1) The more fear the other
person shows, the more likely it is that you will learn a phobia from
watching her, and 2) the more upset, aroused or anxious you were
before watching, the more intense your learned phobia will be.

We are both scuba divers, a sport we enjoy and which, if
approached sensibly, is reasonably safe. We are often asked by
nondivers, "Aren't you afraid of sharks?" The honest answer is "Yes,
if we see one." The truth is that most sports divers rarely see a shark
and even then it's usually just a glimpse. You have more chance of
being hit by lightning than being attacked by a shark, and more
people are killed by bee stings than by sharks. Knowing these facts,
we were struck by how easy it is to learn a phobia when we noticed

how many people became frightened of swimming in the sea after watching the movie *Jaws* and its various sequels.

The third way you can learn a phobia is by simple instruction, by someone repeatedly giving you information about how dangerous something is. You might have never had direct contact with a snake and you might never have seen someone else have a frightening experience with a snake. But someone, possibly with good intentions, tells you repeatedly to be careful in places where there might be snakes. If you do eventually meet a snake, you can be primed to overreact with alarm or panic. It would not be surprising if that became a phobia for you. But it seems possible for people to be "instructed" into a phobia without actually meeting their feared object or situation. If the information (or in many cases the misinformation) creates enough anxiety, apparently that can be enough to give you a phobia.

None of these three possible learning situations will necessarily be enough to give you a phobia instead of just an intense fear. You also need the same elements as in other anxiety problems. That is, the learning experience triggers anxious apprehension about the next possible risky situation. There is a shift in your attention focus, both to your inner anxious reactions and to being overalert for possible risks. You develop the tendency to avoid situations you see as risky. All of this implies that people who learn phobias rather than intense fears probably have the same biological vulnerability to overreacting to alarms that underlies other anxiety problems.

DO DRUGS HELP?

There is nearly universal agreement among researchers, not only about the best psychological plan for treating phobias (which we'll explain shortly), but also that drug treatments do not help, either by themselves or in addition to psychological treatment. If someone has suggested that you use antianxiety drugs to treat your phobia or you have decided to use nonprescription drugs yourself (including alcohol), we strongly advise you to stop using the drug now by working through chapter 3.

MANAGING A SIMPLE PHOBIA

Managing a simple phobia is similar to managing panic problems and agoraphobia, as outlined in the previous chapter, because again the most important ingredient will be to confront your unreasonable fears. We will give you detailed instructions about confronting your fears shortly.

You will feel more confident in your ability to do this if you have some coping skills up your sleeve, so that you feel able to control your reaction. Therefore, your complete plan is to learn how to manage your anxious feelings (work through chapter 10), how to manage your anxious thoughts about your phobia (work through chapter 11), and how to manage the physical components of your anxiety (work through chapter 12). You should go through these chapters before you work on the next section.

CONFRONTING YOUR UNREASONABLE FEARS

You probably won't feel enthusiastic about our suggestion that you need to confront your unreasonable fears to solve your anxiety problem, so let us explain why it is both necessary and usually successful. As we explain in chapter 1, a lot of research into anxiety problems is going on now and there is not yet complete agreement on how the various problems are caused. But it does seem clear that some learning is involved, including learning false alarms, learning to fear your anxiety reactions, and learning to avoid certain situations. We explain above the three ways you might learn a phobia. Similarly, panic problems and agoraphobia involve learning to expect and fear panic attacks in certain situations. Learning, as a cause of unreasonable fears, is also the key to solving them.

A LESSON IN LEARNING

You have almost certainly heard of the pioneering Russian psychologist Ivan Pavlov and his experiments with dogs. Simply, Pavlov noted that when he rang a bell, an untrained dog did not pay much attention. But, as you would expect, if he put some food in the dog's mouth, it salivated. Pavlov then rang the bell at the same time as he delivered the food. After a couple of times doing this, he found that his now trained dog would salivate when he rang the bell alone, without any food. The bell had become a "learned food" for the dog, with much of the capacity of real food to cause the dog to salivate.

Of course, dogs aren't dopey (except ours). Pavlov's dogs quickly realized they couldn't eat the bell. If Pavlov kept ringing the bell without delivering any food at the same time, his dogs would gradually salivate less and less. The learning needed to be reinforced if it was going to be maintained. The process of learning a new stimulus-response link is called *conditioning* and it depends on reinforcement for its occurrence and maintenance. The process of losing the learned stimulus-response link, by not delivering any reinforcement, is called *extinction.* Extinction is usually the most powerful way to remove an unwanted learned behavior; it is much more effective than punishment.

What's the point of this crash course in learning theory? You can see how you might learn to feel frightened of something that is not a real threat, if you experience it at the same time as a real threat. It's not hard to see how false alarms might be learned. But why don't they extinguish? After all, this learning depends on being reinforced if it is to continue. Unless you were in the unusual situation of having a real threat occur most of the times your false alarm occurred, the effectiveness of your false alarm should be fading through extinction. But, as you may have noticed yourself, anxiety problems can be durable. Why?

The answer is simple. Fear is arousing. It activates you to either tackle the threat or escape from it. If you see yourself as unlikely to cope with the threat, you will naturally feel a strong urge to escape, and that's what happens with anxiety problems. In most cases they involve some avoidance of feared situations. By avoiding the situation, you avoid experiencing your learned fear and that's the short-term reward for avoidance. But, by not experiencing your learned fear, there is no chance for it to extinguish. Apart from the cost of the restriction on your life caused by your avoidance habits, they are actually preserving your anxiety problem.

This simple learning theory for unreasonable fears is already being questioned by some research and will undoubtedly be revised and extended in the future. However, it will do for our purposes because it explains why it is necessary to confront an unreasonable fear to get rid of it. Only by actually experiencing your unreasonable fear, without it being reinforced by a real threat, can you extinguish it. We have taken some time to explain this because we want to convince you how important this part of your program will be, even though it will make you uncomfortable. One of the most common reasons for people not solving phobias, panic problems or agoraphobia is that they do not complete this part of their program.

Only by actually experiencing your unreasonable fear, without it being reinforced by a real threat, can you extinguish it.

STRIVING FOR 70 PERCENT

For most of the problems people consult us about, not only anxiety problems, we have to advise that solving the problem will involve some discomfort. Self-defeating avoidance for short-term relief but long-term cost turns out to be a basis for many problems. Gritting your teeth and confronting your problem turns out to be a basis for *solving* many problems. As a rule of thumb, you should aim at confronting your unreasonable fears up to your 70 percent maximum discomfort level.

Imagine the worst you can feel confronting your fear. That's 100 percent. Imagine having no discomfort at all. That's 0 percent. Following our steps below, you will be aiming to confront your fears until you reach the 70 percent level. Then, if you want to, you can leave the situation and calm down. If you want to stay and tough it out for a while at your 70 percent level, that's fine, too. But there is no advantage in going above your 70 percent level.

There are two reasons for this 70 percent rule.

1. It is less unpleasant than going to the 100 percent level, so you are more likely to keep working through this part of your program and less likely to give up.
2. It emphasizes that you are in control of how much you confront your fear and when you take a break from it. One of the major components of anxiety is the feeling of being out of control of your reactions or of the situation. This is an important opportunity for you to learn that you are back in control.

PLAN A GRADUAL APPROACH

This part of your program will require some thought from you. The idea is to figure out a gradual approach to your unreasonable fear, so that you can confront it at your 70 percent level, step by step, until you have defeated it. So ask yourself, what factors about my unreasonable fear make me feel better or worse?

For example, if you were tackling a phobia of dogs, you might decide that the factors affecting how you feel were the size of the dog, how close to you it was, and whether or not it was restrained on a lead or behind a fence. If you were tackling a phobia of heights, you might decide the relevant factors were how high you were, whether or not you could see the ground, and whether there was some sort of barrier between you and the drop. If you were tackling a phobia of traveling in a car, you might decide the relevant factors were how fast the car was going, how busy the traffic was, whether you were the driver or passenger, and whether you could easily turn off the road.

Considering you can develop a phobia for anything, we can't sketch out the ingredients of a gradual approach to every possible phobia. In any case, what makes a difference for you might be different from what matters to someone else. However, there are two common factors that most people can use: time and distance. You can usually gradually increase the amount of time you spend confronting your fear. And you can often gradually increase how close you get to your fear.

Apart from those two common factors, you will need to look at your reactions to your feared situation to identify other relevant factors for you, which you can now gradually change. You don't have to get this dead right the first time. Figure out a plan and try it. If you find there is a factor you missed that makes a big difference in how you feel, revise your plan. A good plan will have about eight to ten steps in it, although you don't have to be rigid about this. Below is an example of a plan for gradually confronting a phobia of riding in elevators.

You can usually gradually increase the amount of time you spend confronting your fear. And you can often gradually increase how close you get to your fear.

As you can see, the relevant factors for this person were how high the elevator was going and whether she was alone or had her husband with her. The other factor she could vary was the amount of time she stayed in the elevator. After she had figured out the possible situations to put in her plan, she then arranged them in order of difficulty for her. She started with the least difficult, Step 1. When she could handle that, she moved on to the next, and so on. She did not wait until she felt no discomfort at a step. That would take too long and it isn't necessary. She moves on as soon as she thinks she will have no more than a 70 percent reaction at the next step. It is essential that you experience your unreasonable fear in order to extinguish it.

It can be difficult to figure out a gradual approach to some phobias. For example, if tackling a phobia of flying, it's hard to arrange for flights of gradually increasing duration. Once you're in a plane, you're probably committed to at least an hour's flight. We once did a project helping women with extreme fears of giving birth. We couldn't tell them to start out having a quarter of a baby! If your phobia is of having injections, you can't have half an injection.

In cases like these, you need to use your imagination. First, you can imagine some aspects of the situation that you can gradually

Plan for Gradually Confronting a Phobia of Riding in Elevators

Step 1   Get into an elevator, accompanied by my husband, without riding up, for one minute, then two, then three, then four.

Step 2   Repeat Step 1, without my husband.

Step 3   Get into elevator, accompanied by my husband, and ride up one floor.

Step 4   Repeat Step 3, without my husband.

Step 5   Get into elevator, accompanied by my husband, and ride up five floors.

Step 6   Repeat Step 5, without my husband.

Step 7   Get into elevator, accompanied by my husband, and ride up ten floors.

Step 8   Repeat Step 7, without my husband.

To get started, this person found an elevator that is not used much. The later steps were done in increasingly busy elevators so that the amount of time the elevator took to reach her floor might be increased by other passengers stopping at intermediate floors. She can also extend her plan by riding up for more than ten floors.

change, such as spending time at the airport or in a labor ward or birthing center. For injection phobias, we advise people to handle syringes and give injections to oranges (which feels just like a person). You can also try to imagine being in your feared situation as vividly as possible. The more realistically you can imagine the situation and your anxious reaction to it, the more your fear will extinguish. If your discomfort gets past the 70 percent level, imagine something pleasant or relaxing until you are ready for another dose. It helps if you also imagine yourself using your new coping skills successfully, after you have imagined how anxious you would feel.

A GRADUAL APPROACH TO PANIC AND AGORAPHOBIA

A gradual approach to agoraphobia isn't too hard to figure out. You might plan to increase how far you travel from home, how long you stay away, how busy the places are you go to and so on. If you have been using a person or something else as a safety signal (see page 56), you must plan to gradually reduce how much you use it, until you do not depend on it at all.

How you plan a gradual approach to panic problems isn't so obvious, but it can be done. The fear of having a panic attack somewhere without support underlies most agoraphobia. So if you are working on agoraphobia, you will need to include steps for dealing with a panic attack. What you are going to do is confront the *symptoms* of having a panic attack so that you learn that they are unpleasant, but not the end of the world—and not out of your control.

Identify the symptoms of a panic attack that are most noticeable to you. Now, figure out how you can practice those symptoms so that you can confront them. If you mostly notice disturbances in your breathing, you can practice them by breathing rapidly. If you mostly notice your heart beating, moderate exercise will make your heartbeat more noticeable. If you mostly notice dizziness or fainting, try turning around quickly on the spot. Do this somewhere where you won't hurt yourself if you fall over, or get a helper to spin you around in a swiveling chair. If you mostly notice tension in your chest (making you fear a panic attack), try tensing the muscles between your ribs. Your personal plan for practicing the symptoms of a panic attack might include several of these methods. You can make the confrontation even more effective if, while practicing the symptoms,

> The fear of having a panic attack somewhere without support underlies most agoraphobia. So if you are working on agoraphobia, you will need to include steps for dealing with a panic attack.

you also imagine yourself in the situations in which you fear having a panic attack.

Sounds unpleasant, even frightening? We sympathize, but we insist. Only by confronting and experiencing your unreasonable fears will you extinguish them. Don't forget, you will take yourself up to only the 70 percent level and you will have some coping skills to keep you in control after you read chapters 10 through 12.

Practical Exercise

Draw up your plan for confronting your unreasonable fear, whether it is a phobia, panic or agoraphobia. Take your time to identify the factors in the situation that make a difference in your level of anxiety. Use your imagination if you need to. Then see if you can figure out ten or so steps of increasing difficulty for you.

Factors that affect my anxiety level:

_____   _____

_____   _____

_____   _____

_____   _____

_____   _____

_____   _____

_____   _____

(continues)

Steps for confronting my phobia:

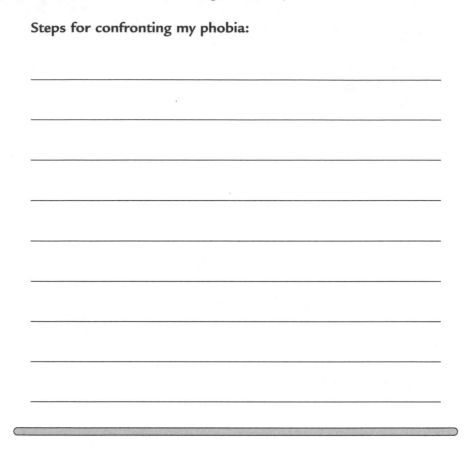

GET SOME HELP

Because you are going to be confronting unpleasant fears and deliberately allowing yourself to reach 70 percent of maximum possible discomfort, you are in for some hard work. Earlier we reported that the most common reason for people not successfully tackling unreasonable fears is that they give up on confronting the fear because it is so unpleasant. Shortly we will give you a suggestion about how you can personally motivate yourself to stick to your plan, but right now we want to encourage you to get some help.

A good helper would be your spouse, a relative or close friend. In fact, many people with unreasonable fears already get help from someone whom they use as a safety signal. "I can go down the street as long as so-and-so is with me." The person used as a safety signal is usually someone who does know about the sufferer's problem and who can offer support if the feared panic attack or phobic object were to arrive. These safety-signal people may disapprove of or not understand the problem, but they give the sufferer a sense of security. Unfortunately, they are actually being used to help the sufferer avoid his unreasonable fear and so, inadvertently, to protect the problem.

We are sure this is not the kind of help they would intend. We have already asked you to plan a gradual withdrawal of any safety signals, as a part of your plan for confronting your fears. So you will need to explain to anyone you have been using as a safety signal that you are weaning yourself off her support. At the same time you can explain that she can now help you in another, very important way, by encouraging you to follow through on your plan to confront your fears and prompting you to use your coping skills.

Research indicates that having your spouse (or some other close support) actively involved with you in this program improves your chances of being successful. So we strongly suggest you get some help, if that's possible. Of course, the amount of help you can get from a relationship is going to depend on how supportive that relationship is. Few people confronting unreasonable fears do better without involving their spouses, because their marriages are already strained. What do you think? If it's clear your marriage is having problems, we encourage you to do something constructive about that, such as seeing a counselor together. If you don't think your marriage is necessarily troubled, but you and your spouse aren't too sure how to be supportive, work on the communication skills in chapter 13.

> Research indicates that having your spouse (or some other close support) actively involved with you in this program improves your chances of being successful.

Ask your helper to read at least this chapter. Show him your plan for gradually confronting your fears and explain the coping skills you are going to use (see chapters 10, 11 and 12). Then explain that you would appreciate his encouragement to keep you working through your plan. Be careful what you ask for. Do not use your helper as a safety signal who always accompanies you when you confront your fears. Do ask your helper to provide encouragement and assistance in your attempts to confront your fears. If you need to have your helper accompany you to get started, make sure you deliberately plan to gradually reduce your dependence on him.

STICKING TO DIFFICULT GOALS

We often help people work on goals that they know are in their own interests and that they want to achieve, but they can see that reaching these goals will be difficult. Sticking to an exercise program or a study plan or quitting smoking are common examples. There is a well-tested technique you can use to strengthen your motivation in such situations. You can write a motivational contract. This is simply a promise you make to yourself to work consistently on your plan for confronting your fears and not avoiding them. Below is an example of a motivational contract for confronting fears. This one is for the person who drew up our earlier plan for confronting her phobia of riding in elevators (see page 75). She has decided to work on her plan at least three times a week. That's not bad. The more you can practice, the faster your progress will be.

Motivational Contract for Confronting a Phobia

Each week, my plan for confronting my fear of riding in elevators includes at least three half-hour practice sessions. I will reward myself with (for example) a new book (or a treat or access to a fun activity or money into a special reward account). For any week that I don't do this, without a genuine excuse, my penalty will be (for example) doing a chore (or missing out on a fun activity or donating the amount I use as a reward to a charity).

    I realize this contract is a motivational aid I am using to help me stick to a plan that I know is in my own best interest. So, if I cheat on it, I am only cheating myself.

Sign and date your contract and put it up somewhere where it can act as a reminder. If you are using a helper, he can sign it, too, as a witness, and help you to keep track of your practice sessions and decide whether you have earned your reward or your penalty.

Practical Exercise

If you have not yet worked through chapters 10, 11 and 12, you should do those now so that you have a good set of coping skills to help you confront your fears. If you have been using antianxiety drugs to treat your fears, we strongly encourage you to work through chapter 3 now. Is there someone you are going to ask for help in carrying through your plan to confront your fears? Do you and he need to strengthen your communication skills? How? Will it help you to stick to your plan if you write yourself a motivational contract? Try a rough draft in the spaces below, then when you're ready, get started.

My motivational contract:

_____

_____

_____

_____

_____

_____

A SPECIAL TIP FOR BLOOD OR INJECTION PHOBIAS

A blood phobia involves, as you would guess, an intense fear of the sight of blood. It can be a problem if it causes you to overreact to even minor wounds or necessary medical treatment. It can also stop people from being blood donors, which is a pity. Your blood is the one organ you can donate to someone in need, over and over again, because your body replaces it. We won't digress into a lecture, but donating your blood is a socially worthy activity open to most of us. Make some regular deposits in your local blood bank and you won't feel any guilt about making a withdrawal, if you ever need one.

The general idea of a blood phobia involves excessive fears of any surgical or medical procedure, when those fears can result in your fainting. This can include receiving minor surgery, such as stitches in a cut, dental treatment, or receiving an injection. People can often avoid such phobias until, for example, they need vaccinations for a trip overseas. We have had some people come to see us for their injection phobias just before they're due to leave. Our best advice then is to postpone the trip! If you don't want to wind up in that situation, tackle your injection phobia now. If you only feel anxious about these events and therefore try to avoid them, the instructions above are for you. If your anxiety about these events makes you likely to faint, you will need the additional suggestions below.

What is unusual about a blood phobia is that it is the only phobia that causes its victims to faint. You will remember that fear is an arousing reaction, activating you to deal with the threat. But a blood phobia seems to contradict this because it can cause you to become so deactivated that you pass out. This apparent puzzle has now been solved. Dr. L. Ost, an active Swedish researcher of phobias, has found that people with blood phobia do have the usual activating reaction to their feared stimulus (in that research, watching a film of surgery), including marked increases in heart rate and blood pressure. However, this was followed by marked decreases in heart rate and blood pressure. Since this lessens the blood supply to your brain, you may then feel dizzy, nauseated and faint.

It is interesting that people with blood phobia do not faint in other frightening situations and people with other kinds of phobias do not faint when in their feared situations. We don't know why blood phobia has this unusual effect but it is possible that it is a primitive defense reaction. If the blood you were fainting at was your own, because you had a serious wound, lowering your heart rate and blood pressure could reduce your bleeding.

In any case, it means there is an important variation in managing blood phobias as opposed to other phobias. You will use increased muscle tension to counteract the fainting tendency. By tensing the large muscles in your arms, legs and body, you can push your blood pressure back up and prevent yourself from fainting. Practice to get the hang of this and then start the same gradual approach to your unreasonable fear as outlined above. For approaching situations involving blood, you may need to use photographs, movies or your imagination.

For an injection phobia, you can buy or borrow several syringes and needles of different sizes and practice giving injections to an orange, as we suggested earlier, but imagining as vividly as you can that it is you getting the injections, not the orange. (Chefs and cooking fans note: Keep your largest syringe and needle in the kitchen and use it for injecting wine or some other basting liquid into your meat dishes. Who said psychology couldn't be fun?) Dr. Ost has developed a treatment for injection phobias, using a gradual approach in one long consultation, by the end of which the patient is taking his own blood sample (rather than making an injection). Naturally, you should only try this procedure with the help of a cooperative and supportive doctor or nurse who can make certain you are taking all necessary precautions against infection and so on. But, if you want to try it, we can tell you we have seen it done and it works! It's a good idea to try your practice sessions lying down, then sitting, so that you won't hurt yourself if you do faint. But aim to be able to stand up eventually. Then you might visit your local blood bank!

7

Social Phobia and
Social Anxiety

- A social phobia is an excessive fear not just of being with others but of being evaluated by others.
- Focusing on your anxiety distracts you from the task and lowers your performance.
- It is usually restricted to one or a few situations, unlike shyness and general social anxiety.
- Social phobics tend not to have associated problems, although some will panic in their phobic situations.
- Socially anxious people often lack social skills and do tend to have other associated problems.
- Solving a social phobia requires changing your unrealistic thoughts about and confronting your feared situations.
- Solving shyness and social anxiety involves strengthening social and interpersonal skills and confronting social situations.
- Drugs, including the beta-blocker drugs, have not been proven helpful for social phobia or anxiety.

A *social phobia* is an excessive fear, not just of being with other people but of being assessed by other people. So it occurs in situations where you are required to do something while others may be observing and, you believe, judging your performance. As with other anxiety problems, it involves shifting your attention away from the real task and onto your anxiety reactions, both your physiological arousal and your negative expectations of how you will be judged. This shift in attention causes a drop in your ability to perform, confirming your fears and increasing your anxiety.

The most common social phobia seems to be of public speaking. Other common examples include meeting people, eating in front of others, signing your name in front of others, social mixing or conversations, or urinating in public toilets. A social phobia that haunts many students is exam phobia, although it is not restricted to examination situations. Any assessment situation, such as making a presentation to a class or study group, can bring out the phobia. Knowing that a written assignment will eventually be assessed can be sufficient to elicit the phobia and stop the student from completing the assignment, maybe even from starting it.

Social phobias are common, affecting about 2 percent of the population. It isn't clear whether they affect men or women more. They tend to begin in late adolescence or early adulthood. It is probably no coincidence that many people are most performance-conscious at this stage of life.

SOCIAL PHOBIA VERSUS SOCIAL ANXIETY AND SHYNESS

A social phobia is not the same as shyness, although people with a social phobia may act shyly in order to avoid their phobic situation. Shyness tends to be a more general social anxiety. A shy person feels uncomfortable in most, if not all, social situations. Many shy people lack some common social skills. There is a particular problem that probably represents the extreme of shyness, called an *avoidant personality*. Someone with this problem is extremely sensitive to rejection or humiliation. He reacts very strongly to even a hint of disapproval and can only cope with relationships that are uncritically accepting. He usually has few, if any, friendships.

A social phobia is not the same as shyness, although people with a social phobia may act shyly in order to avoid their phobic situation.

The *Diagnostic and Statistical Manual* defines social phobia as much more restricted, usually limited only to specific situations, although one person may have several such phobic situations. People with social phobia may handle most of life quite well, including other social situations, and do not usually lack social skills. They don't always avoid their phobic situation but may develop techniques for toughing it out instead. Even then, they report feeling anxious while in the situation. Sometimes famous people, such as TV and radio performers, movie stars and sports stars, suffer from social phobias. They will usually keep up the job—"the show must go on"—and may keep up appearances, although often their performance does actually suffer.

What clearly pinpoints a social phobia is that the person usually has no difficulty performing the task, whatever it is, in private. It is the presence of an audience that throws them. There are several other points that distinguish social phobia from shyness and general social anxiety. Social phobias usually develop suddenly, from your teens on. Shyness and social anxiety tend to be present from childhood, sometimes getting gradually worse. People with social phobia only occasionally have other associated problems. People with social anxiety often have marked associated problems.

What clearly pinpoints a social phobia is that the person usually has no difficulty performing the task, whatever it is, in private. It is the presence of an audience that throws them.

Although a few people may suffer from both social phobia and social anxiety, it does seem that these are two different problems, resulting from different causes. Some research suggests that extreme shyness, at least, has a strong genetic component. This does not mean that, if your problem seems more like extreme shyness than social phobia, you are stuck with it. It does mean that you need to learn to live with it and to manage it.

Practical Exercise

Can you decide whether your problem is social phobia or general social anxiety (shyness)? Try this checklist:

Social phobia	Shyness/social anxiety
Sudden onset, from teens on	Problem since childhood, maybe gradually worsening
Restricted to one or a few specific situations	A problem in most or all social situations
Probably no associated problems	Probably associated problems, maybe marked
Focuses on fear of being judged	Often reflects a lack of social skills

---

IF YOUR PROBLEM IS SOCIAL ANXIETY

If your problem seems more likely to be shyness and general social anxiety, you can begin to work through chapters 10 and 11 now. If you are aware of strong physical signs of anxiety in social situations, you should also work through chapter 12.

If your social anxiety has led you to avoid social situations, you will need to confront those next, in a gradual way. See chapter 6 for the steps for gradually confronting a feared situation. If you think your social anxiety reflects a lack of social skills, you should next work through chapter 13, and you might find chapter 14 helpful, too. If that all seems like a lot, you're right, it is. You might reasonably expect to take several months to work through all of those chapters and the rest of your life to polish up some of your coping and social skills. So the sooner you get started, the better!

On the other hand, if you think your problem is social phobia rather than shyness and general social anxiety, we have further information for you. Read on.

WHAT CAUSES SOCIAL PHOBIA?

Social phobias can seem like a puzzling problem. They often occur in people who were previously fine and who still function well in the rest of their lives. They can seem "silly." You can sign your name or urinate in a public bathroom (or do whatever the task is) perfectly well in private, so why does it suddenly become difficult when someone else is present? Swedish psychologists have come up with an interesting theory about social phobia.

In chapter 1 we point out that fear is normal in humans and other animals and it can be adaptive, activating us to react to an apparent threat. So, these psychologists believe, we are prepared by our evolutionary history to fear certain wild animals because these animals threaten our lives. It certainly would be an advantage to humans if they *automatically* feared animals such as lions and tigers without having to find out the hard way what a threat they can be.

Humans are social beings. We usually live and work with other humans. Being able to relate successfully to others plays an important role in personal success and health. So, the theory goes, humans may be prepared by our evolutionary history to fear social threats, such as anger, criticism or rejection, *automatically*. For example, these researchers trained volunteer subjects to be frightened by some pictures of faces. Some of the faces looked angry, some neutral and some happy. It was found that the learned fear continued to be associated with the angry faces while it faded away from the neutral and happy faces.

There seems to be something special about an angry face that causes it to be more easily associated with fear. This effect even depended on where the eyes in the face were looking. A picture of an angry face looking away lost its learned fearfulness just as a happy or neutral one did. It was a picture of an angry face looking at you that retained its fearfulness. This ties in with observations of our near relatives, the other primates such as chimpanzees and gorillas, for whom direct eye contact is often associated with aggression and fear.

So it seems that we humans may be naturally sensitive to anything we associate with social criticism or rejection. This may well be the particular biological vulnerability that leaves us open to developing social phobia rather than some other anxiety problem.

This would explain why social phobia centers on an unreasonable fear of having your performance of a particular task judged critically by someone else. It is the exaggerated fear of not doing the task well, and therefore of being criticized or rejected, that triggers the anxiety process. As in other anxiety problems, the sufferer then shifts her attention away from the task and onto her anxious reactions. This shift in attention can make the fear a self-fulfilling prediction, as her performance does decline and the whole problem feeds on itself. Some people can sit in an exam situation, too petrified to write anything, for hours.

> So it seems that we humans may be naturally sensitive to anything we associate with social criticism or rejection.

SOCIAL PHOBIA AND IMPOTENCE

Professor Barlow has an intriguing theory that the common male sexual problem of erection difficulty (often called *impotence*) is a particular example of social phobia. Certainly a similar process is involved. In most cases we find that the man initially suffers some difficulty with his erection for quite understandable reasons, such as illness, fatigue, stress or drugs. However, he either does not recognize this cause or does not see it as a sufficient explanation for his sexual difficulty. He often believes he has failed, especially to satisfy his partner, and fears her criticism or rejection. On the next sexual occasion, he worries about failing again and shifts his attention away from relaxing and enjoying his sexuality onto anything that suggests he is about to have difficulty with his erection. Not paying attention to the relevant sexual stimuli in the situation is enough to interfere with his erection response. As soon as he notices this reduction in his "performance," he worries more and his attention shifts even further. As a result, his anxiety and his erection difficulty both increase.

This theory fits quite well with our own explanation of erection problems and it is interesting that our program for solving these problems is just what you would expect from Professor Barlow's theory. If you think you are anxious in social or sexual situations because you are not confident about your sexual skills, you will find some helpful suggestions in chapter 13.

DO DRUGS HELP?

There has been little research into the usefulness of the usual antianxiety or antidepressant drugs in treating social phobia. Given the strong evidence of risks associated with the antianxiety drugs and the negative side-effects of the antidepressant drugs, there would seem to be no good reason, then, for using these drugs to treat social phobia. If you have been prescribed these drugs, we encourage you now to wean yourself off them (see chapter 3).

In recent years, nevertheless, there has been a peculiar fad for drug treatment of social phobia, using a group of drugs called *beta-blockers* (this name just refers to how the drugs affect particular nerve cells). The strange thing about beta-blockers is that they have usually been prescribed to treat high blood pressure and sometimes migraine headaches. Why should such drugs help with social phobia? No one knows and, when you look carefully at the evidence, they may not really help at all.

A careful review of eleven research studies found that in eight, beta-blockers did seem to help more than a placebo in reducing performance anxiety. None of those eight studies were done with people who would meet the diagnostic rules for having a social phobia. Rather, the subjects were ordinary people facing an anxiety-provoking performance situation such as a bowling competition, an exam, public speaking or a public musical performance. In each case, the drug was given just before the performance.

This one-time use is quite different than the regular use a genuine social phobic would require because he has a more marked problem and usually has to confront his fear frequently. The only preliminary research with genuine social phobics found beta-blockers to be no help. Professor Barlow noted that the three studies of the eleven above that showed no positive effect were studies that didn't involve musicians. His hunch was that the beta-blockers, if they were having a beneficial effect at all, were not reducing performance anxiety as such but might be reducing anxious trembling in the fingers. This in turn would improve musical performance.

Recently, the U.S. Food and Drug Administration approved Paxil (paroxetine—an SSRI) specifically for treating social phobia. This drug is not without its side effects, most notably fatigue, tics, agitation, apathy, memory problems, drug-induced Parkinsonism and—most disturbing for many—sexual dysfunction. These are only the side effects revealed over the past decade. This drug has not been studied for long enough to reveal side effects that appear decades after use. Only recently have reports of brain damage, disfiguring tardive dyskinesia and symptoms resembling muscular dystrophy began to surface.

At present, the available research favors psychological treatment over drug treatment for social phobias. There is simply no evidence yet that any drugs offer worthwhile, lasting help with social phobia. This includes the drug that many men will resort to: alcohol. Your performance is not improved by drinking alcohol. It only diminishes your ability to critically appraise your performance.

MANAGING SOCIAL PHOBIA

There are two main components of a program for managing a social phobia: changing your thoughts about the situation and confronting the situation. The instructions for changing your thoughts are given in detail in chapter 11. There are several common features in the thoughts associated with social phobia. We suggest you take some time to check your self-talk, as explained in chapter 11, to see which of these apply to you.

People with social phobia often have unrealistic ideas about how much attention others will pay to them and how easily others will notice any signs of anxiety or any drop in performance, no matter how small. They often set themselves impossibly high performance standards, seeing anything other than a perfect, error-free performance as a failure. And they often have unrealistically disastrous expectations of the consequences of not performing to these perfect standards. They especially expect to be judged negatively by their "audience" and they tell themselves this judgment is very important.

> People with social phobia often have unrealistic ideas about how much attention others will pay to them and how easily others will notice any signs of anxiety or any drop in performance, no matter how small.

Well, did that list ring any bells? Are there other thoughts you have about your social phobia situation? Chapter 11 explains how to test these thoughts and replace them with more realistic ones that do not cause you unnecessary anxiety. You should also learn the coping strategy in chapter 10. When you say the coping statement to yourself while confronting your social phobia situation, it will be important for you to remind yourself to focus your attention on the task at hand and not let it wander onto your anxious reactions.

The instructions for confronting fearful situations in chapter 6 will also be helpful to you. Applying those instructions to a social phobia, however, may require two important variations. First, you may not be able to figure out a gradual approach, as we have suggested people do when confronting a simple phobia. For example, you can gradually increase how long you stay in and how far up you ride an elevator, because that's entirely under your control. But for a social phobia of, say, writing your name in front of someone else, you either do it or you don't.

A gradual approach may not be as important for confronting a social phobia, anyway, so don't worry if you can't figure one out. You can always use your imagination, as we suggested in chapter 6. Imagine yourself in your phobic situation for gradually increasing amounts of time. Make sure you imagine your anxious feelings as realistically as you can, then imagine yourself using your coping skills successfully. Don't make it too easy for yourself. Imagine some of the things you fear might go wrong and then imagine how you will cope with those.

If you have social phobias for several situations, you can use them to make a gradual approach. Rank them in order of their difficulty for you and start by confronting the least difficult. When you can handle that one—remember the 70 percent rule from chapter 6—then confront the next one and so on, until you have tackled all of your social phobia situations.

The second point about confronting social phobias is an important one. You will remember that in the definition of a social phobia we said that some people will not avoid their feared situations but will instead have worked out ways for toughing it out. To meet the definition of a social phobia, there must be a strong urge to escape from or avoid the situation, but you won't necessarily act on that urge. Usually your performance is suffering because of your distracting anxiety reactions, but you're still going into the situation.

In fact, this causes confusion for some people with social phobias. When they are told that an important part of their treatment is to confront their feared situations, they reply, apparently accurately, "But I don't avoid the situation. I go into it often and that hasn't helped me at all. How is going into it again supposed to help me now?"

What psychologists have found is that some people are *internal avoiders,* meaning that they physically go into their feared situations but psychologically avoid them. Some people do this by distracting themselves in some way; some pretend they are somewhere else; others avoid participating in the situation. For example, you may sit in a group (such as a class) but avoid saying anything. This internal avoidance protects you from the full possible anxiety in the situation and so, as we explained in chapter 6, protects that anxiety from extinguishing.

Some people are *internal avoiders,* meaning that they physically go into their feared situations but psychologically avoid them.

The practical implication of this is that you must involve yourself fully in the feared situation that you are confronting. If you have been coping with the situation by avoiding it psychologically, you must now stop that avoidance and let yourself experience your anxiety about the situation so that it can extinguish. Don't distract yourself, don't pretend you're somewhere else, focus on the task at hand. If that makes you uncomfortable, use the coping skills in chapters 10 and 12.

A PRACTICE AUDIENCE

If you consult a qualified clinical psychologist about a social phobia, she may suggest that you take part in a group therapy program. Although many people are initially embarrassed by the idea of discussing their personal problems with a group of strangers, there are two advantages to a properly conducted group-therapy program for social phobia (as distinct from a simple cost-cutting, unstructured group meeting). As with other problems, it can help you to feel less alienated to hear that other people are facing difficulties like yours and you can support each other's attempts to solve these problems.

Particularly for social phobias, it can be helpful to get others to simulate your feared situation. In a proper group-therapy program, this will be arranged for you. But in a self-help program, you might still arrange it for yourself. If your social phobia is public speaking of some sort, can you ask a small number of family or friends to be the audience for some practice runs? If your social phobia is signing your name in front of someone, can you ask just one other person to be your practice audience? Even if it would be initially embarrassing to ask for help, especially for a social phobia like using public bathrooms, that will be less of a price to pay than being stuck with your phobia. Ask your assistants to read this chapter and maybe chapter 6, describe the feared situation you are asking help with simulating, and give it a try.

SOCIAL PHOBIA AND PANIC

Finally, to manage your social phobia, you may need to do something about managing panic. It is not unusual for people with social phobia to panic in their feared situations. It is sometimes difficult at first for us to decide whether someone coming in for treatment has a panic problem or social phobia. The key to distinguishing between these problems is to look carefully at the situations in which you have (or fear) panic attacks. If the situations are ones in which you expect to be evaluated by others, then you have social phobia. If the situations are ones that take you away from "safe" places or people, then you have a panic problem.

For example, people with social phobias often have no problem being alone in public places. Their panic attacks tend to be restricted to the situation or situations in which they believe their performance is being assessed by someone. They are often most concerned about having signs of anxiety that others might notice, such as blushing or perspiring. On the other hand,

> People with social phobias often have no problem being alone in public places. Their panic attacks tend to be restricted to the situation or situations in which they believe their performance is being assessed by someone.

people with panic problems tend to have problems in a wider range of situations and are more concerned with reactions that signal a possible panic attack.

For our purposes, we don't need to draw a hard line between panic and social phobia. It's enough to recommend that, if your social phobia includes panic attacks, you will need to learn to manage them, too, from chapters 5 and 6.

Practical Exercise

What now? Take the following steps, depending on your situation.

1. If you have decided your problem is social phobia, you should now work through chapter 11 to begin tackling your unrealistic fears of being judged negatively.

2. Then work through the instructions in chapter 6 for confronting your feared situations, bearing in mind our suggestions in this chapter.

3. If confrontation is going to make you feel anxious, prepare yourself by working through chapter 10.

4. If you tend to be distracted by the physical signs of your anxiety, work through chapter 12.

5. If your social phobia has caused you to panic (or fear you are about to panic), work through chapter 5.

6. If strengthening your social or sexual skills will help you confront your feared situations, work through chapter 13 and, if strengthening your interpersonal skills will help, work through chapter 14.

7. If you have been using drugs because of your social phobia, we strongly encourage you to work through chapter 3.

Once again, that's a good few months worth of steady work. You will need to use some of your coping skills for the rest of your life. But that still beats having social phobia interfere with living.

8

Posttraumatic Stress Disorder

- A posttraumatic stress disorder (PTSD) is an anxiety problem that can occur after a life crisis, which is any event causing unusually strong emotional reactions.
- The Crisis Response and Recovery Cycle describes how people normally react to a crisis.
- Most crisis victims do recover, depending on their resources, the intensity of the crisis and the availability of support.
- Crisis victims who are vulnerable to anxiety may develop a PTSD.
- A PTSD is marked by 1) experiencing the event over and over again; 2) avoidance of anything associated with the crisis; 3) avoidance of any strong feelings, through reduced involvement in activities and relationships; and 4) signs of increased anxiety since the crisis.

- The core of a PTSD is a fear of being overwhelmed by the strong feelings associated with the crisis. Managing a PTSD involves confronting this fear by not avoiding but instead confronting reminders of your crisis experience, with the aid of several coping skills and preferably some support.

Posttraumatic stress disorder is a bit of a mouthful, so we'll abbreviate it to PTSD and explain what it means. We don't like jargon and try to avoid using it, but there is no simple, commonly used word or phrase that covers the idea of PTSD.

Problems such as *shell shock, combat fatigue* and *war neurosis* are some better-known examples of PTSD, but these labels imply the problem is peculiar to victims of war. Unfortunately, it seems possible for a PTSD to occur in a vulnerable person who is the victim of any life crisis, not only of war. So we'll use the term "PTSD" and try to make sense of it for you. Since PTSD is a problem that may occur after traumatic stress, let's begin with that.

TRAUMATIC STRESS AND LIFE CRISES

We define a *life crisis* as any event that causes you to experience unusually strong emotional reactions that have the potential to interfere with your ability to function, at the time or later. To cause such unusually strong emotional reactions, a typical crisis is itself an unusual event, at least in any one person's life. In fact, the psychologists' guidelines in the *Diagnostic and Statistical Manual* for defining PTSD begin with the person "having experienced an event that is outside the range of usual human

> Unfortunately, it seems possible for a PTSD to occur in a vulnerable person who is the victim of any life crisis, not only of war.

experience and that would be markedly distressing to almost anyone."

Some of the life crises that could obviously lead to PTSD include

- a personal disaster, such as a violent crime, assault or rape
- a life-threatening experience or illness
- the death of someone close
- a large-scale disaster, such as fire, flood or a large accident.

Less obvious but just as possible triggers include

If your reaction to a situation is strong enough to interfere with your ability to function normally, at the time or afterward, then that situation is a crisis for you, regardless of whether it would be a crisis for someone else.

- family crises, such as incest, abuse or discovering your spouse is having an affair
- life-stage crises, such as losing your job or having to relocate

Some psychologists might argue that these events are not unusual enough to meet the *Diagnostic and Statistical Manual* rules, but we think that misses the point.

In our self-help book for people trying to cope with a life crisis, *Surviving: Coping with a Life Crisis,* we emphasize that the defining characteristic of a crisis is the degree of emotional reaction it causes in you. It is the need to cope with these unusually strong emotional and associated reactions that constitutes the "traumatic stress" in PTSD. Stress is the process of coping with the demands in your life. Your strong feelings in reaction to a life crisis are themselves a further demand on your coping skills, a "traumatic" demand because they are sudden and potentially harmful.

If your reaction to a situation is strong enough to interfere with your ability to function normally, at the time or afterward, then that situation is a crisis for you, regardless of whether it would be a crisis for someone else. If you are vulnerable and if you don't receive adequate support at the time or soon after, then your crisis may trigger a PTSD for you, regardless of whether it has that effect on someone else who experienced the same crisis.

THE CRISIS RESPONSE AND RECOVERY CYCLE

In *Surviving: Coping with a Life Crisis*, we describe the way people usually react to and then recover from a crisis. Before we outline that here, however, we want to emphasize that the Crisis Response and Recovery Cycle is a description of the *average* way in which people react. It is not a prescription for how you should or must react if you are "normal." It is truly normal for all humans to differ from each other. We are similar, but not identical. So your crisis reaction and recovery will be similar to this description, but not necessarily identical, and that makes you normal.

The Crisis Response and Recovery Cycle (CRRC)

1. Crisis response

   - Shock
   - Disbelief
   - Realization
   - Non-emotional survival state

2. Release or escape

3. Recovery cycle

   - Shock
   - Depression
   - Mood swings
   - Anger
   - Philosophical reflection
   - Laying to rest

THE CRISIS RESPONSE

The *crisis response* is your immediate reaction to the actual crisis, so it lasts as long as the crisis does. It typically begins with shock, because a victim will usually have been going about her normal daily life when the crisis occurred or began. It is the unexpected nature of crises that gives them much of their emotional impact.

> Just as the physiological shock reaction is a primitive defense reaction by your body, disbelief may be a simple attempt to protect yourself psychologically.

Shock.   The physiology of shock causes noticeable physical symptoms:

- a white face
- nausea
- dizziness, perhaps fainting
- fast and shallow breathing
- fast heart rate

If the situation is very frightening, the person may lose control over his bladder or bowel. While this is often the subject of sneering jokes, you should understand that these are involuntary responses caused by the overwhelming stimulation of the crisis and not by any lack of nerve or courage.

Disbelief.   Because crises are unusual and unexpected events, part of your reaction may be disbelief: "This can't really be happening, not to me." It is possible that this disbelief is also a way for your mind to buffer itself against the full impact of the crisis. Just as the physiological shock reaction is a primitive defense reaction by your body, disbelief may be a simple attempt to protect yourself psychologically.

Realization.   As the crisis continues, the disbelief gives way to the realization that the situation is real, not imaginary or a joke. This acceptance of the reality of the crisis may increase the level of shock. In any but a very brief crisis, it usually leads to the fourth component of the crisis response, a non-emotional survival state.

Non-emotional survival state.   In this state, a victim's emotions become frozen and flat. Many people remark after a crisis that they are surprised how calm they (and others) were during the crisis but, in fact, this is the most common reaction. There are two popular but misleading ideas about how people react to a crisis.

1. The heroic myths depicted in adventure movies show the hero cleverly and fearlessly escaping from the threat. A few people do act bravely and resourcefully during or, more often, immediately after a crisis, usually people who have had some special training for dealing with emergencies. Most people don't; they freeze. Later, they may feel unnecessarily guilty for not reacting more bravely or usefully during the crisis.
2. The panic myths from Hollywood disaster movies show crisis victims running around screaming. A few people do panic in this way, usually people who were vulnerable to panic anyway. Most people don't; they freeze.

In chapter 1 we describe freezing as a normal part of an intense fear reaction in many animals. If your threat is a predator about to attack you, freezing may be adaptive in not drawing attention to you or not inviting further attack.

Of course, if your threat is not a predator, freezing may be no help or may prevent you from taking useful action. These are primitive reactions, ingrained, automatic, and not necessarily helpful. This is true also of your thinking in this frozen state. While it focuses narrowly on your immediate survival, which could be adaptive, it can be so narrow that you don't think of helpful actions that later may seem obvious. Again, crisis victims may later make themselves feel unnecessarily guilty for not thinking more clearly during the crisis.

This non-emotional survival state usually lasts for the rest of the crisis reaction, ending when there is a release or escape from the crisis itself. In the case of a long-term crisis, such as coping with a long, possibly terminal illness in yourself or someone close, there are usually times when you temporarily escape from the crisis by being involved in other activities, slipping back into the non-emotional survival state when you have to go back and confront the crisis again.

RECOVERY

Most people do recover from their crisis experiences, although this may take anywhere from days to months, depending on the severity of the crisis, the amount of social or professional support they receive, and their own psychological resources or vulnerability. There have been varying estimates of, and some debate over, how many crisis victims suffer a PTSD, but a careful look at the research suggests that this apparent variability is largely explained by the factors just listed.

A higher proportion of victims of an intense crisis will be at risk of PTSD than will victims of a less intense crisis. Social support and post-crisis counseling can both aid recovery and reduce the risk of PTSD, possibilities we will return to. The better a person's coping skills, the more likely she is to cope and recover. And there is accumulating evidence that victims of PTSD show the same biological vulnerability to anxiety found in other anxiety problems, a vulnerability that is brought out in their case by their crisis experience.

Shock. The recovery stage usually begins with shock again, lasting from a few hours to several days, depending on the severity of the crisis. This period of shock is often marked by dull, flat emotions. While this may insulate the victim from some of the impact of his crisis, it is often misinterpreted by others as meaning that the victim is not very distressed. They may unwisely encourage this illusion with well-intended but quite inappropriate reassurances such as "Forget it, now that it's over." This is about the worst advice you could ever give a crisis victim because it encourages denial of their normal reactions. This denial in turn can become the avoidance that characterizes PTSD.

Depression.   After the initial shock of escape, many victims experience depression, an understandable reaction to their "bad luck." While depressed, there is the risk that a victim will withdraw within herself, breaking off contact with family or friends and losing valuable emotional support. A breakdown in important relationships can become a part of later PTSD. This risk is worsened by the fact that some people avoid contact with a crisis victim, partly to protect their own feelings, and possibly because they feel unable to help the victim.

Mood swings.   Towards the end of their depressive phase, many victims have marked mood swings, up one day but down the next. Seeing his emotional state as unpredictable and out of control can cause anxiety for the victim. This is exactly the fear that plays a central role in anxiety problems, including PTSD. These mood swings can also confuse and worry family and friends, possibly further isolating the victim.

Anger.   Most crisis victims will experience anger, again an understandable if unpleasant reaction to what has happened to them. This does show that the victim is working through her recovery, and anger is a change from being a passive victim to trying to grapple with the world again. However, it can have negative consequences if not handled skillfully. If your anger cannot be directed toward the real cause of your crisis, you may misdirect it toward family or friends, adding to your isolation. If you feel guilty about your unreasonable anger, you may slip into denying your feelings again.

> Anger is a change from being a passive victim to trying to grapple with the world again. However, it can have negative consequences if not handled skillfully.

Philosophical reflection. Crisis victims usually spend some time in philosophical reflection, replaying their experience in their minds, trying to make sense of it. This reliving of the crisis can be unpleasant and, in excess, self-defeating. But some reflection is normal. Essentially the victim is trying to explain to himself why he suffered his crisis, because then he may be able to protect himself against a repeat experience. Even if he has to conclude that it was due to extremely bad luck, he may then be able to believe that it's unlikely to happen again.

Laying to rest. If you work through a successful recovery from a crisis experience, you will eventually lay it to rest, as a bad memory that does not intrude too much into your present life. You may feel you have been changed in some ways by your experience, and you may feel briefly uncomfortable if you are reminded of it, but it does not interfere significantly with your normal functioning. This is quite different from PTSD.

If you decide that your present problem is really that you are still working through a crisis response or recovery, as we have just described it, you should find *Surviving: Coping with a Life Crisis* helpful. It is focused on the CRRC and includes practical suggestions for the family, friends and associates of crisis victims. These people are often upset by the victim's apparent distress but don't know what to do to help. Sometimes they mistakenly encourage victims to deny their quite normal bad feelings. *Surviving* offers suggestions for avoiding mistakes like that while giving potentially important support to the victim.

WHAT IS PTSD?

As we said above, the psychologists' rules for defining a PTSD begin with the person having experienced an unusual event that would be distressing for almost anyone. However, we emphasize again that what defines a life crisis is not how common it may be, but the strength of your emotional reaction to it.

The second characteristic of PTSD is that the person keeps experiencing the crisis event over and over again, in one or more of the following ways.

- You may have recurring distressing memories of the event. This is different from the philosophical reflection that normally occurs during crisis recovery, intended to make sense of the event. These memories are unwanted, intrusive and seem out of your control.
- Young children may repetitively play out the theme or some aspects of the event.
- You may have recurring dreams of the event. These are also distressing and can disturb your sleep.
- You may suddenly feel you are having the experience again. These flashback episodes can be vivid and are often accompanied by perspiration, trembling, heart palpitations and shortness of breath, symptoms you will note are very like those of a panic attack.
- You may feel distressed by something that to you symbolizes or resembles the event. A common example is the anniversary of the crisis.

The third characteristic of PTSD, as with other anxiety problems, is avoidance—in this case, avoidance of reminders of the event or of your feelings:

- You may not be able to remember important aspects of the event.
- You may avoid situations that remind you of the event, even though these are situations you need or want to go into.
- You may show generally reduced emotional responses, such as a loss of interest in previously significant activities and a feeling of detachment from other people, including those who were close to you.
- You may believe your future is unlikely to be successful.
- Young children may slip back in their development; for example, losing language or toilet skills.

The fourth and final characteristic of PTSD is that your level of arousal has been persistently higher since the crisis. This may be indicated by at least two of the following symptoms:

- difficulty sleeping
- irritability or outbursts of anger
- difficulty concentrating
- heightened sensitivity to stimulation
- inclination to overreact when startled
- physiological reactions, such as sweating, when exposed to something that reminds you of the crisis

To decide that a patient has PTSD, a psychologist will check that the characteristic symptoms listed above have been happening for at least a month. He will also probably check if it was more than six months after the event that the symptoms began, but that need not concern you now for your self-help project.

WHAT CAUSES PTSD?

It is not enough to say that having a life crisis causes PTSD, because many people do recover from a crisis without developing a PTSD, especially if the crisis was not too severe, if they receive social or professional support, or if they had good coping skills already.

There is growing evidence that people who develop a PTSD after a crisis experience were already vulnerable because of a biological tendency to overreact to threats. This is the same vulnerability that seems to be involved in other anxiety problems and recent research is finding the same sort of family history of anxiety problems in people with PTSD as in people with other anxiety problems.

> There is growing evidence that people who develop a PTSD after a crisis experience were already vulnerable because of a biological tendency to overreact to threats.

Professor Barlow has concluded that the explanation for PTSD, then, may be much the same as for phobias. During her crisis experience, a person already vulnerable to anxiety is likely to have a strong emotional reaction, which is traumatic in itself. She is also likely to see her reaction as abnormally bad and out of her control. After the crisis is over, instead of working through a recovery as we described it above, she is frightened of the possibility of her extreme bad feelings occurring again. This would explain the avoidance that marks PTSD, whether it is avoiding anything she sees as related to her crisis or avoiding any strong feelings at all. Just as someone with a panic problem actually fears another panic attack, someone with PTSD fears a recurrence of the strong feelings associated with the past crisis. These feelings are seen as unpredictable and out of her control, as are the anxious reactions in other anxiety problems. This would account for the intrusive and upsetting nature of memories, dreams and flashbacks of the crisis.

This explanation for PTSD makes a lot of sense to us and it also suggests strongly what will be necessary to successfully solve a PTSD, which we will outline shortly. But first, what about drug treatments?

DO DRUGS HELP?

There have been no properly conducted, scientific evaluations of drug treatment of PTSD yet, although there are a few case studies claiming that antidepressant drugs were helpful and antianxiety drugs less so. Given the possible side effects and problems involved with these drugs, we have to conclude again that we cannot recommend drug treatment for PTSD. If you have been using drugs to manage your PTSD, we suggest you work through chapter 3.

This advice also applies to self-prescribed drugs, including alcohol and tobacco. There is a tragically high amount of drug dependence, including on alcohol and nicotine, among people with PTSD.

MANAGING PTSD

Since the basic mechanism in PTSD seems to be a learned fear of strong emotional reactions, just as a phobia is a learned fear, the basic treatment is the same: Confront your fears. It will help you to create and understand your treatment plan if you read chapter 6 now. As we have explained there, you will feel more confident about confronting your fears if you have some coping skills to help you manage your reactions.

The central fear in a PTSD is that you are going to suffer strong emotional reactions that are out of your control. So it makes sense now to prove to yourself that you will be in control. You will feel bad when you confront your fears. As we explain in chapter 6, that's necessary if your fears are ever going to fade. But you don't have to feel overwhelmed. Working through chapter 10 will help you manage your anxious feelings. Working through chapter 11 will help you manage your anxious thoughts. Working through chapter 12 will help you manage the physical symptoms of your anxiety. Then you are ready to confront your fears.

We describe the basic plan for confronting unreasonable fears in chapter 6, but keep in mind the following important points about applying that plan to PTSD. First, the fear you are setting out to confront is the fear that you cannot cope with your reactions to your crisis, that you will be overwhelmed by feelings out of your control if you let yourself be reminded of it. So confrontation requires that you do let yourself be reminded of your crisis.

In fact, the various treatments for PTSD that have been developed over the years are mostly variations on this theme. For example, this was the basis of *abreaction,* the therapy developed for treating war neuroses during World War II. A similar approach was successfully developed more recently for Israeli soldiers during the Lebanon conflict.

CONFRONTING BAD MEMORIES

We'll illustrate this plan with two examples. One is a woman who has developed PTSD after being in a bad car crash, the other a man who developed his PTSD after being in a naval accident in which a ship sank and many sailors drowned. Both are examples of real people who have consulted us.

Try to identify the reminders that you have been avoiding. These could be situations that resemble the original bad experience. For example, she could only travel in a car if she was driving, not as a passenger, and not in fast-moving traffic. He would feel so uncomfortable below decks—"Where escape might be difficult"—

that he eventually resigned from the navy, which had been his career in life. He even quit a later job on a small, youth-training ship for the same reason. Notice how their avoidance was saving them from feeling anxious but at the price of big restrictions on life.

Avoided reminders can be situations that might prompt memories of the original bad experience rather than being like the experience themselves. For example, her car crash happened on the way to her lawn bowls club, when she had taken a ride with two of her friends from the club. So she was avoiding going to the bowls club in case she met one of those friends or anyone who might ask her about the accident. Likewise, he stayed away from veterans' clubs for years in case someone asked him about his navy experiences. Again, both were achieving short-term anxiety avoidance at long-term cost.

Or, the reminders may be actual memories of the original event or associated feelings. She would turn off the TV news if it was about a car accident. He refused to talk about his bad experience, even with his wife, adult children, or close friends, even when they were trying to understand how his PTSD was affecting their relationships. She avoided strong emotions by leading a restricted life and taking the drugs she got her doctor to prescribe for her. He avoided strong emotions by drinking excessively.

Often the reminders are dreams, or rather nightmares, in which you relive the bad experience. Sometimes the dreams are so bad that the PTSD sufferer fears going to sleep unless he has taken enough drugs, of whatever kind, hopefully to keep the nightmares away or unconscious. This is a sad situation, and if it applies to you, you owe it to yourself to work on a better solution. Keep going.

Make a list of the reminders you have been avoiding. Situations resembling your original bad experience? Other situations in which you might be reminded of the experience? Memories of the experience? Situations that might trigger emotions that in turn remind you of the experience? Sleeping without drugs? For each one, note how you have been avoiding it, because you are going to stop that.

Now, following the guidelines in chapter 6 for gradually confronting unreasonable fears, work out your plan for gradually confronting the reminders you have been avoiding. For example, she was able gradually to increase the distance she traveled in a car as a passenger, the speed of the traffic she would drive in, the amount of time she spent at the bowls club, and how much she told other people about her accident. she also weaned herself off her antianxiety drugs (see chapter 3). He was able gradually to increase how much he told his family about his bad experience, then the amount of time he spent at a veterans' club and how much he told his friends there about his experience. He cut back his drinking to a much healthier level, with encouragement from his wife.

So far, you will notice these two people were tackling avoidance behaviors they could stop and replace with more successful behaviors. The problem with dreams and nightmares is that they are not voluntary behaviors, so you can't just choose to stop them. Don't worry, that wasn't the point of this exercise. We are encouraging you to stop *avoiding* reminders. We are *not* saying that you won't always have some reminders, but you can expect that they will happen less often and trouble you less. Get this goal and expectation clear. Intrusive dreams, nightmares or flashbacks are the symptoms of your PTSD problem. As you solve that problem working through this program, those symptoms should gradually get less frequent of their own accord. That's something to look forward to. Meanwhile, if you have been using drugs of any sort to avoid bad dreams, nightmares, or flashbacks, we suggest you now wean yourself off those drugs. They are not your long-term answer.

Use your anxiety-management skills when you confront your back memories (see chapters 10, 11, and 12). Have these skills ready, up your mental sleeve, as you work through the steps above. Confronting your bad memories instead of avoiding them will be unpleasant enough; you don't have to do it cold turkey. For example, you could apply the coping statement from chapter 10 like this:

I expect to feel bad when I let myself remember my bad experience because that's how it would affect anyone. I can cope with those natural bad feelings and trying to avoid them has cost me too much. It is not a sign of weakness or incompetence or craziness that I feel bad when I have those memories, it's a sign of being human. I'm not going to dwell on what happened to me, that's just rubbing salt in the wounds. But I also won't avoid being reminded by doing things that cost me more in the long term than the temporary relief is worth. Now, what do I want to do next, regardless of whether or not it brings up some bad memories?

And find your answer to that question, give yourself a shove in the back, and do it.

Yes, it is much easier for us to suggest this plan to you than it will be for you to do it, at least at first. But it beats being stuck with a PTSD problem and its side effects. If you expect to have trouble sticking to your plan, take a look at our suggestions in chapter 6 and below for getting help from others and for helping yourself to stick to a difficult plan.

DO YOU NEED TO RELIVE YOUR BAD EXPERIENCE?

For a long time, the standard treatment for PTSD problems involved helping the sufferer to relive, in her imagination, her original bad experience. There is no doubt that this procedure helped many people to break their avoidance habits and confront their bad memories and so to work through them and get them into a better perspective. However, as you would expect, this was usually a very unpleasant procedure, especially because it typically involved helping her to relive the experience as vividly as possible. Recently the need to relive the original experience has been questioned for two reasons. First, if you can solve your PTSD problem by following the steps above without having to relive all the details of the original experience, that's going to be less unpleasant for you and you are less likely to give up on the project. Second, there is some concern that a vivid reliving of a traumatic experience may be traumatic itself. If the original bad experience didn't get you, maybe reliving it vividly will. There is already some evidence of this happening when PTSD sufferers have been treated by overzealous but poorly trained counselors, especially in some self-help groups.

So, do you need to relive your original bad experience if you are going to successfully lay it to rest? Well, that's how you decide, by seeing if you can lay your bad memories to rest rather than try to avoid them. We suggest you first work carefully through the steps above, using the coping skills in chapters 10, 11 and 12 to help you. We believe that will be sufficient for many PTSD sufferers and can see no good reason for suggesting you give yourself a harder task than you already face. Give yourself a well-earned pat on the back if that turns out successfully for you. This would mean that, whenever life reminds you of your bad experience, you will feel bad temporarily, maybe say the coping statement to yourself, and then get on with life without any unreasonable, self-imposed restrictions. Well done.

On the other hand, if you do try the steps above and they have not been enough to achieve a successful solution as we have just described it, you can then add the more powerful but demanding procedure of reliving your original crisis. You may also need to do this if you have been so good at avoiding reminders that you can't identify many to tackle in the way we described above. So you will need to use remembering the original experience as your way of confronting bad memories. No, this is not pleasant, but it is effective. You can help yourself to manage your reactions and stay in control if you have first mastered the skills recommended above.

USE YOUR IMAGINATION

It is usually not practical, let alone safe, for people to relive a crisis experience in reality. Confronting a crisis experience is usually done by imagining the experience again.

1. Find a comfortable and private place, where you can count on not being disturbed.
2. Relax yourself as much as you can, although you will naturally feel tense about what you are about to do.
3. Then try to remember your crisis as vividly as you can.
4. If your anxious reactions—feelings, thoughts or physiology—become strong, use your coping skills to manage them. But notice the emphasis is on *managing* them, not trying to deny them. You are out to prove to yourself that you can cope with your natural reactions to your crisis.

Jog Your Memory

We point out above that one form of avoidance people with PTSD engage in is to blot out their memories of their crisis experience. This can mean that you now have difficulty remembering important parts of what happened, which naturally makes it difficult for you to relive the experience. See what you can find to jog your memory. Anything that you can associate with your crisis will do, such as photographs, diagrams, news reports, talking to others who were there, maybe returning to the scene.

A technique some people find helpful is called *elaborated writing*. Sit down and write out a description of your crisis. Use your own memories and any other sources of information available. When you have finished, go back to the beginning and write it again, trying to add more detail to each sentence. You might try to get only the bare facts into the first version. Next time, try to add some description about what you could see, hear, smell or touch. Then try to add more detail about how you felt and what you thought. Gradually you will build up a more vivid description and, in the process, relive it more realistically.

_____

_____

_____

_____

_____

TAKE YOUR TIME

Psychologists treating people for PTSD have found that you need a reasonably long time of imagining the crisis before your fears of not coping begin to fade. At least thirty minutes and up to sixty minutes seems to work best. Perhaps people need this much time to overcome the barriers they have been hiding behind and to prove that they really can cope with their reactions.

Dr. Mardi Horowitz is a recognized expert in this field. He believes that it is important to adopt a gradual approach to confronting a PTSD. Although there is no research evidence yet to show that a gradual approach is more effective than a head-on approach, it is obviously less unpleasant and it may help you to stick to your plan. You could plan a gradual approach, either by varying how much time you spend or by varying the intensity of your experience. Remember the suggestion in chapter 6 of aiming to confront your fears up to 70 percent of the worst possible reaction.

GET SUPPORT

We have referred to the evidence that social or professional support can help people to recover from a crisis and so prevent the development of a PTSD. In *Surviving: Coping with a Life Crisis,* we explain to family, friends and associates how they can provide valuable support to a crisis victim. The same possibility applies here. If you have been suffering from a PTSD, there is a strong risk that your important relationships have suffered. It will help them and you if you now ask some of those people, important in your life, to read at least this chapter so that they understand what has happened to you and what you are doing about it.

It will help you to carry out your difficult confrontation program if you can get some support for that, too. For this purpose, you might approach just one or two people to help. Ask him, her or them to read this chapter and, preferably, chapter 6 as well. Explain to your helper what your coping skills are and how you intend to use them to manage your reactions to reliving your crisis. This is important because your helper's task is to encourage you to use those skills and to confront your fears, not to feel distressed when you get upset and then encourage you to quit.

IF THE DAM BREAKS

If you have had the clamps on your feelings, strictly avoiding any reminders of your crisis, don't be surprised if, at some point while confronting your fears, a strong emotional reaction pours out of you, like water from a broken dam. This can be sudden and dramatic, possibly frightening you or your helper. However unpleasant this is, it is an important breakthrough that you will eventually welcome. The intensity of this reaction just shows you how much feeling you have had bottled up all this time.

Since your goal is to prove to yourself that you can manage your reactions to your crisis, even the strongest ones, neither you nor your helper should be tempted to quit too soon. Within our 70 percent guideline, keep yourself in confrontation with your crisis and give your fears a chance to fade. If you find this too difficult for self-help, then it's time to get some professional help from a clinical psychologist or other trained counselor. It is not time to hide from your crisis experience again.

Practical Exercise

If you have not yet worked through chapters 10, 11 and 12, you should do so now so that you have a good set of coping skills to help you confront your PTSD. If you have been using drugs, prescribed or otherwise, to manage your PTSD, we strongly encourage you to work through chapter 3 now. Are there people important to you who also need to learn about your PTSD? Are you going to ask someone to help you confront your

PTSD? Do you need a motivational contract to help you stick to your plan? In the space below, write out your plan for reliving your experience and confronting your memories, then get started.

What factors make facing reminders of my experience better or worse? (Number them in order of most difficult.)

_____   _____

_____   _____

_____   _____

_____   _____

_____

Using your list above and the Jog Your Memory exercise (see page 116), write out your plan for gradually confronting your fears, in steps (see the sample step-by-step plan on page 75).

_____   _____

_____   _____

_____   _____

_____   _____

_____   _____

9

Obsessive-Compulsive Problems

- Obsessions are thoughts that persistently intrude into your mind, making you anxious.
- The most common obsessions are about dirt, contamination, aggression, violence, sex, religion and physical illness.
- Compulsions are behaviors you feel compelled to do over and over, to protect you from the threat that your obsession is about. They can be actions or thoughts. The two most common are excessive cleaning and checking.
- Obsessive-compulsive problems are often associated with depression that, if more than mild, should also be treated.
- We cannot recommend drug treatment for obsessive-compulsive problems.
- Managing an obsessive-compulsive problem involves confronting your fears about the obsessional thoughts and preventing the compulsive behaviors.
- You will probably need some coping skills and support to do this successfully.

Obsessions are thoughts that persistently intrude into your mind, making you anxious. Compulsions are behaviors that you feel compelled to do over and over, to protect you from the threat that your obsession is about. Notice their relationship to each other. Obsessive thoughts increase your anxiety while compulsive acts are intended to decrease it. For example, repeatedly thinking that your hands have been contaminated by germs may lead to your repeatedly washing them.

It used to be thought that obsessive-compulsive problems were rare, but a survey by the American National Institute of Mental Health, published in 1984, found that 1 to 2 percent of the general population suffered from this problem. While that figure may seem low, it means millions of unhappy people when applied to the whole population and it makes obsessive-compulsive problems almost twice as common as panic problems. These problems are often associated with depression and can be difficult to treat successfully, so this frequency is of some concern.

Obsessive-compulsive problems usually begin in late adolescence or young adulthood, like most other anxiety problems, but they can occur in children as young as five or six, worrying their families, and in adults as old as fifty. They seem to be more common in women than in men. For example, one study found that 80 percent of people with a problem of compulsive washing were women, although again we wonder if that reflects the cultural practice of women doing most of the washing.

WHAT IS AN OBSESSION?

According to the guidelines in the *Diagnostic and Statistical Manual*, *obsessions* are persistent ideas, thoughts, impulses or images that the person sees, at least initially, as intrusive and senseless. Because these intrusive thoughts make him anxious, he will try to avoid them, as happens with other anxiety problems. He may try to ignore or block them or to neutralize them with a compulsive behavior. Although he

> Obsessive thoughts increase your anxiety while compulsive acts are intended to decrease it.

sees these thoughts as intrusive, he does recognize them as the product of his own mind, not as something being imposed from outside. This is an important point because it distinguishes between obsessive-compulsive problems and other psychological problems such as schizophrenia, in which the sufferer believes his intrusive thoughts are being put into his mind by someone or something else. This book is not intended for those kinds of problems.

The most common obsessional thoughts are about one or more of the following:

- dirt and contamination
- aggression and violence
- sex
- religion
- physical illness

But people can become obsessed with any fear or doubt, no matter how logically unlikely it may be. Many sufferers will have more than one obsession. In extreme cases, people may spend a lot of their time dwelling on their obsessive thoughts, suffering extreme anxiety, depression and guilt.

Yet psychologists have found that obsessional thoughts are apparently quite common. In studies comparing people with obsessive-compulsive problems to people with no anxiety problems, they found that both groups reported having some obsessional thoughts, about similar topics and with similar discomfort that would prompt them to try to resist the thoughts. The differences were that the people with problems had more frequent obsessive thoughts, found them less acceptable, experienced more intense anxiety about them and tried harder to resist them. The point about this is that it seems some obsessive thoughts may be a fairly common event, especially when your stress level is up, with the potential for becoming a problem. We will come back to this point.

WHAT IS NOT AN OBSESSION?

In daily conversation we will sometimes talk about someone being "obsessed" with something, meaning that she spends a lot of time and energy on it. While this may reflect an imbalanced lifestyle, it is not necessarily an obsession of the kind we are concerned with here. In an extreme form, this preoccupation is called an *overvalued idea.* This is an isolated belief that the person has strong feelings about and closely identifies with. You will notice the difference from a true obsession, which causes discomfort and anxiety from which the sufferer tries to escape. An overvalued idea may seem strange to others but it is something the person values and *chooses* to be preoccupied with.

> The difference between these worrying thoughts and obsessional ones is in their content and how you feel about them.

It is also important to distinguish between obsessional thoughts and just plain worrying. In chapter 1 we point out that worrying is a normal part of anxiety and that it can be adaptive. Anticipating possible problems and their consequences can prompt you to do some constructive preparation and therefore help you to cope if the problem arises. If anxiety is becoming a problem, like the general anxiety problems described in chapter 4, you are likely to find yourself worrying more. The difference between these worrying thoughts and obsessional ones is in their content and how you feel about them.

First, the worrying thoughts associated with general anxiety problems may become repetitive and intrusive but they tend to reflect the current problems in your life, even if they are exaggerated. In contrast, obsessional thoughts are usually recognizably improbable. Second, people with general anxiety want to worry because they see it as a necessary part of defending themselves against their anticipated threats. People with obsessional thoughts do not want them because they make them feel anxious. It is the thoughts themselves that are the threat in an obsessional problem.

Obsessive or Worried?

Can you now decide whether you are troubled by obsessive thoughts, as we have defined them? This would mean that your intrusive thoughts are

- repetitive and persistent
- the product of your own mind
- a cause of discomfort and anxiety to you
- something you try to resist, by blocking them out, ignoring them or doing a repetitive action

If your intrusive thoughts don't fit this pattern, or if you can't decide, it may be time to get some professional help.

WHAT IS A COMPULSION?

According to the guidelines in the *Diagnostic and Statistical Manual,* compulsions are repetitive, purposeful and intentional behaviors done in response to an obsession. They are done according to a set of rules or in a stereotyped way, making them like rituals. Compulsive behaviors are intended to neutralize the threat represented by the preceding obsession or to lessen the discomfort caused by the obsession. The person acting compulsively recognizes that his behavior is unreasonable but that recognition is not enough to stop it. Sometimes it even makes him feel worse about the compulsive behavior.

The two most common forms of compulsive behavior are excessive cleaning and checking. The obsessional fears of excessive washers tend to focus on the risk of being contaminated by some object or situation. Their excessive washing is then intended to restore safety and a sense of control. The obsessional fears of checkers tend to focus on possible threats or disasters. Their excessive checking is then intended to prevent the imagined threat or disaster.

> Some people will develop compulsive thoughts rather than actions. These are repetitive and ritualized thoughts that occur in the same way and serve the same purpose as compulsive behavior.

However, just as obsessional thoughts can develop around anything you might see as a threat, compulsive behaviors can take any form that you might see as protecting you from that threat. In particular, some people will develop compulsive thoughts rather than actions. These are repetitive and ritualized thoughts that occur in the same way and serve the same purpose as compulsive behavior. Common examples of compulsive thoughts are "magical" words or phrases and prayers. In this case, there is no outwardly observable sign of the compulsive part of the problem because it is being done in the person's mind. Some people will have a number of compulsive behaviors, sometimes both actions and thoughts.

WHAT IS NOT A COMPULSION?

Sometimes a compulsion becomes so entrenched in a person's behavior that it can become a habit, no longer closely associated with her level of anxiety. It seems that it was once used to ward off the anxiety caused by an obsession but, with lots of use, it becomes a habit in itself. Researchers have called these *rituals*. It is useful to identify them because, since they are no longer tied to an obsession, they are treated differently.

It is also necessary to distinguish compulsions from a much less common problem called *primary obsessional slowness*. In this problem, the person does seem to be behaving in a ritualized way but instead is behaving very slowly, as though acting in slow motion. One case involved a patient who took four hours to get up each morning. It was clear that this was different from obsessive-compulsive behavior because it was not accompanied by intrusive, unpleasant thoughts or strongly negative feelings. He was slow, not because he had repetitive behaviors, but because he had divided each behavior, such as washing his face, into many little steps that he did very carefully.

Primary obsessional slowness is therefore unlikely to be an anxiety problem and our plan below is not suitable for it. It may be the extreme of what people commonly call an "obsessive-compulsive personality." This is the kind of person who is generally thought to be excessively orderly, neat, clean or conscientious. In fact, there is no evidence that this kind of person is any more likely than anybody else to develop an obsessive-compulsive problem. Further, their apparently "obsessive" behavior is quite different from the problem we are describing here, because it is neither compulsive nor accompanied by much emotion.

Just as many apparently normal people report some obsessional thoughts, so they also report some apparently compulsive behaviors. For example, one study of college students found that 10 to 15 percent of them reported excessive checking, far more people than we would expect to have an obsessive-compulsive problem. When the psychologists compared frequent checkers who did not have an obsessive-compulsive problem with students who did not check things frequently, they found the checkers tended to have poorer memories and were generally more depressed and anxious. It is reasonable to conclude that checking things is a normal and possibly adaptive behavior that is increased by increased stress and has the potential to become a problem. Again, we will return to this point.

Are You Compulsive?

Can you now decide whether or not you are troubled by compulsive behaviors, as we have defined them? This would mean that your troublesome behaviors are

- repetitive, maybe following a set of rules, or ritualized
- probably done in response to obsessional thoughts
- intended to protect you from the threat in those thoughts, or to lessen your anxiety about those thoughts

- actions or thoughts you choose to do or think, even though you recognize that they are unreasonable

If your troublesome behaviors don't fit this pattern, or you can't decide, it may be time to get some professional help.

WHAT CAUSES OBSESSIVE-COMPULSIVE PROBLEMS?

By now you may have realized that we are going to suggest that the cause of obsessive-compulsive problems is similar to that of other anxiety problems. Intrusive thoughts apparently occur in most people, particularly when their stress levels go up, and the usual reactions to these thoughts are discomfort and, therefore, attempts to resist the thoughts. For most people, this is no more than a passing problem. But for those who are vulnerable to overreacting to stress, the group who are vulnerable to all anxiety problems, this can begin the development of a serious problem.

It now seems likely that people who develop obsessional thoughts, rather than some other anxiety problem, have previously learned that some thoughts are "dangerous" or unacceptable. Some people consider that thinking of an unacceptable act is as immoral and unacceptable as doing the act. It does seem that, for an intrusive thought to cause significant distress, it has to be personally meaningful or relevant to the thinker. Vulnerable people overreact to the threatening thoughts and this, in turn, sparks strong attempts to resist those thoughts. These attempts will become their compulsive behaviors, either actions or further thoughts.

There is now some evidence to suggest that the form the compulsive behaviors takes also reflects previous experience. One study found that the mothers of compulsive checkers were significantly more concerned about details and more demanding than were the mothers of compulsive washers. Another study found that the parents of obsessive-compulsive patients had emphasized cleanliness and perfection.

The person worries about having more obsessional thoughts and comes to see them as out of her control and occurring unpredictably. This increases her anxiety and stress further, thus making intrusive thoughts even more likely to occur. The compulsive behaviors developed in defense may temporarily reduce the immediate anxiety, but her awareness of the unreasonableness of her behavior ultimately increases her stress. This narrowing focus onto your fears and your reactions to them and the way the problem feeds back into itself are, as you now know, characteristic of anxiety problems.

There is a particular point in this explanation that may account for why obsessive-compulsive problems can be so troublesome and difficult to treat. We have pointed out that these problems develop in much the same way as do other anxiety problems, but there is one key difference. If you have developed a phobia for, say, riding in elevators, then you can at least manage that by avoiding elevators. This may be a major inconvenience if you work on the 23rd floor, but you can at least regain some control. If you have developed a fear of having panic attacks away from your home, you can at least stay home. This will be a major restriction on your life, but you can regain some control.

But what do you do if your fear is not of an object or a situation that you can avoid, but a thought inside your mind? That's not so easy to avoid. When we are helping people deal with intrusive thoughts of all kinds, we make the point that you can't really stop an unwanted thought from beginning. It's like watching a movie you have seen before. You need to see at least a few seconds of it before you recognize it. Similarly, a sufferer's obsessive thoughts have to begin before he can try to resist them with his compulsive behavior. It's not surprising that obsessive-compulsive problems can take over a person's life, with disastrous consequences.

OBSESSIVE-COMPULSIVE PROBLEMS AND DEPRESSION

There is a sadly high overlap between obsessive-compulsive problems and depression; up to 80 percent of patients with obsessive-compulsive problems are also depressed. Most of them are at least mildly depressed; some are seriously depressed. Why this is so, we don't yet know for sure. In chapter 1, we discuss the similarities and differences between anxiety and depression. Professor Barlow believes that they are two different ways of responding to stress in vulnerable people and that whether you become anxious or depressed depends on how vulnerable you are, how severe your stress is and what kind of coping skills you typically use.

It is quite possible that obsessive-compulsive problems cause depression because, as we explained above, the sufferer cannot even regain the limited control over her problem that is possible over some other anxiety problems, if at some cost. This is likely to cause feelings of helplessness and hopelessness, both common components of depression. Such feelings will be reinforced if the sufferer has been given ineffective and inappropriate treatment, as we often find. It is also possible that, in at least some cases, depression first triggers intrusive thoughts that then become obsessional in vulnerable people. For our purposes, we don't need to decide between these possible explanations for the overlap between obsessive-compulsiveness and depression. But we do need to note it, for two reasons. First, depression is a potentially serious problem in itself. If you are significantly depressed, you should be

> When we are helping people deal with intrusive thoughts of all kinds, we make the point that you can't really stop an unwanted thought from beginning. It's like watching a movie you have seen before. You need to see at least a few seconds of it before you recognize it.

doing something constructive about it. Second, there is evidence that depression interferes with some of the steps you will need to take to solve your obsessive-compulsive problem. That's another good reason for doing something constructive, if you are significantly depressed, at the same time as you tackle your obsessive-compulsive problem, if not before.

Practical Exercise

Can you decide whether or not you are depressed, at least depressed enough to need to tackle your depression as well as an anxiety problem? Try this checklist to find out.

_ Do you feel sad, low or blue most of the time?
_ Are you doing much less than you used to?
_ Do you get along with others worse than you used to?
_ Do you feel guilty most of the time?
_ Do you see your problems as too big or hard to solve?
_ Do you doubt that things will ever improve?
_ Are you having trouble sleeping?
_ Do you feel fatigued most of the time?
_ Is your appetite less than it used to be?
_ Have you lost interest in sex?
_ Do you think of suicide?

The more times you answered "Yes," the more likely it is you have a problem with depression and the more desirable it is that you do something constructive about it. It is time to seek some professional help from a clinical psychologist or similarly trained professional.

DO DRUGS HELP?

There is no proper scientific evidence that drugs, prescribed or social, are of lasting help with obsessive-compulsive problems. There is no evidence to suggest that anti-anxiety drugs help at all. So, if you have had these prescribed for an obsessive-compulsive problem, we suggest you wean yourself off them (see chapter 3). There have been some clinical claims that certain antidepressants are helpful and some enthusiastic claims that they are particularly helpful. Unfortunately, this enthusiasm appears to be at the very least premature. For example, one long-term study found that the apparently beneficial effect of one antidepression drug had disappeared when the patients were followed up after treatment. Given the overlap between depression and obsessive-compulsive problems, it would not be surprising if reducing some patients' depression also helped with their obsessive-compulsive problems.

Current research shows that all of the antidepression drugs are about equally effective in reducing depression, including the newer ones, and that they are about as effective in the short term as evidence-based psychotherapy (cognitive-behavioral therapy or interpersonal therapy). As we have already pointed out regarding anxiety, the risk in using drugs to manage your depression is that you may come to believe you need them forever, whereas most depressed people do not. This belief can be reinforced by the fact that most people who successfully used a drug to manage their depression will relapse into being depressed again, after they stop taking the drug. This is because the drugs are really only addressing the symptoms of your depression, no the cause. If drugs, including antidepression drugs, help you over a rough patch in life, that's fine. But we strongly advise you to see them as a temporary aid while you solve the causes of your depression. If one of the main reasons you are depressed now is your obsessive-compulsive problem, then we encourage you to work through our program and solve that problem. That should make you much less depressed.

MANAGING OBSESSIVE-COMPULSIVE PROBLEMS

An obsessive-compulsive problem usually has the two components, obsessive thoughts that cause anxiety and compulsive behaviors intended to counter the thoughts and the anxiety. So your plan for managing an obsessive-compulsive problem needs to tackle both components of the problem. There is good evidence that tackling just one, when both parts are involved, is not effective.

Obsessional thoughts act as anxiety-producing threats, in much the same way as phobic objects or situations do. So the main way you will tackle your obsessional thoughts is also the same, by confronting your unreasonable fears about having those thoughts. Chapter 6 details the basic plan for confronting unreasonable fears. It will help you to plan and understand this part of your program if you read chapter 6 now. You will feel more confident about confronting your fears about your obsessional thoughts if you have strengthened your coping skills (see chapters 10, 11 and 12). You are aiming to prove to yourself that you can have intrusive thoughts and manage the anxiety they cause, without anything disastrous happening. So it will be important that you do allow your obsessional thoughts into your mind.

> Obsessional thoughts act as anxiety-producing threats, in much the same way as phobic objects or situations do.

This means that you must not try to block the obsessional thoughts in any way. That is the second main component of your program, to prevent your compulsive behaviors. This is going to be hard on you. Your compulsive behavior has been your way of protecting yourself from anxiety caused by your obsessional thoughts. So, preventing yourself from doing the compulsive behavior means you will experience that anxiety. That will be unpleasant but, as you will learn from chapter 6, it is only by experiencing that anxiety that you can make it fade. Again, you are going to handle this better if you have already learned the coping skills in chapters 10, 11 and 12.

With those skills up your sleeve, you are then ready to confront your obsessional thoughts and prevent your compulsive behaviors. For example, if your obsessional thoughts have been fears of contaminating your family with germs after you have handled dirty objects and your compulsive behavior has been excessive washing, your goal now is to let yourself imagine being contaminated but stop yourself from any excessive washing. If this makes you feel anxious, use the skills in chapter 10 to manage your feelings. The skills in chapter 11 will help you question your obsessional thoughts (but not block them). If you become physically anxious, use the skills in chapter 12.

DON'T MAKE IT TOO HARD

This will be an unpleasant process, but don't make it too hard for yourself or you may give up. Remember our suggestion in chapter 6 of aiming to confront unreasonable fears up to a level of discomfort of 70 percent of what you imagine would be maximum. For example, you might deliberately rub some dirt on your hands and leave it there until you reach your 70 percent level. Then wash it off and give yourself a break, as well as a pat on the back for tackling a difficult problem. A gradual approach can help you feel in control and not overwhelmed, but make sure you keep making progress.

DO YOU NEED SOME HELP?

We have mentioned that obsessive-compulsive problems can be difficult to solve, not to make you pessimistic, but to alert you to the fact that you will probably need to arrange some support for your program. This could be particularly true for preventing your compulsive behavior. Sometimes this is so ingrained that it takes a round-the-clock watch to prevent it and some patients need the level of support that only a hospital can provide. If preventing your compulsive behavior is going to be difficult, we suggest you try to get help from one or two assistants.

These relatives or friends should read this chapter and chapter 6, at least, so that they understand what you are doing and why and how they can help. For example, you may ask your assistants to hold your hands firmly to stop you from any unnecessary washing. They need to know that this is going to make you feel anxious and that this is necessary for the treatment to work. They can help by suggesting you use your coping skills. They won't help if they encourage you to quit.

PREVENTING RITUALS

Sometimes compulsive behaviors can become so habitual that they become detached from any obsessional thoughts and associated anxiety. In this case, the compulsive rituals won't be preceded by any noticeable obsessional thoughts or increase in your anxiety, but their repetitive occurrence is the problem. There is obviously no need for you to confront any obsessional thoughts, because there don't seem to be any. You can try preventing yourself from carrying out the ritual and see how you feel. If that causes you much anxiety or distress, you will find the coping skills in chapters 10, 11 and 12 helpful.

You can also try some direct approaches to eliminating the ritual. Figure out how long it usually is between each ritual, then try to steadily increase that time. Write yourself a motivational contract (see page 80) for increasing the time between rituals. You can also try scheduling your ritual, in much the same way as we described above for scheduling intrusive thoughts. Because these rituals are habitual and not associated with significant anxiety, it is easy to do them almost unconsciously. In that case, we suggest you ask an assistant to keep an eye on you and, whenever you start a ritual, immediately prompt you to prevent it.

PREVENTING COMPULSIVE THOUGHTS

As we discuss earlier, some people develop compulsive thoughts rather than actions. They are intended, like the actions, to neutralize the threat in your obsessional thoughts, but they are thoughts themselves. They might be words or images; for example, a woman who has obsessional thoughts of harming her child might counter them by imagining the child well and happy. Compulsive thoughts are trickier to prevent because they are all in your mind, so no one else can really help. An assistant might hold your hands to stop you from washing unnecessarily, but he can't "hold" your mind to stop it from thinking compulsive thoughts.

Notice carefully the distinction you have to draw here. You need to admit your obsessional thoughts—the ones that make you anxious—to your mind so that you can confront them. Your compulsive thoughts are the ones you use to counter the obsessional ones that you want to prevent. If necessary, write out all the thoughts (including words, phrases and images) involved in your problem and use your feelings to classify them. The ones that make you anxious are obsessions and need to be experienced to confront them. The ones you have been using to reduce your anxiety are the compulsions and need to be prevented so that you can learn that you don't need them.

Thought-Stopping.   Intrusive thoughts are a common problem and a technique called *thought-stopping* has been developed to help you stop them. When you are confronting your obsessional thoughts and using your coping skills to manage your anxiety, allow those thoughts to continue (at least to your 70 percent discomfort level). As soon as a compulsive thought begins, jump up and shout to yourself, "Stop!" Then go back to thinking your obsessional thoughts or using your coping skills. When a compulsive thought begins again, repeat the procedure.

Yes, this is a bit dramatic and it's obviously a technique you will use in private, or with an assistant who understands what you're doing and can encourage you to stick with it. It is its dramatic impact that interrupts the habitual nature of your compulsive behavior, restoring your voluntary control. If you need to prevent compulsive thoughts when there are other people around, you may be understandably reluctant to shout out loud, but you can do it inside your head. Many people find it helps to wear a rubberband around a wrist, just tight enough to fit comfortably. When you shout or think "Stop," give yourself a sharp twang on the wrist. The small, sudden hurt involved again serves to break the habitual nature of your compulsive thoughts.

Schedule Your Obsessive Thoughts.   Another way in which some people have found that they can regain control over their thoughts is to schedule them. If you estimated that now you spend, say, a quarter of your waking time on your obsessional thoughts and compulsive reactions, you can start with a schedule that allows you to spend 15 minutes having your obsessional thoughts, beginning on the hour every hour. While you do, try to prevent your compulsive behavior, whether actions or thoughts. For the rest of the hour, if intrusive thoughts begin, you tell yourself that you are not allowed to have them until the next scheduled time and try to concentrate on your normal activities instead. Many people have been surprised how much control they can establish over thoughts that they had seen as out of control.

DO YOU NEED PROFESSIONAL HELP?

We don't mean to jinx your self-help efforts—far from it. We would like to encourage you to give self-help a good try, if you believe you can tackle it. There is at least one promising report of a psychologist achieving a good success rate helping people to manage obsessive-compulsive problems, giving her patients lots of homework assignments like our suggestions above. But we accept the evidence that these are harder to solve than many other anxiety problems, especially for people who are also very depressed. If you try self-help and it doesn't work, or if it seems too much to begin, then we encourage you to consult a qualified clinical psychologist or other trained counselor who can help you through a program like the one above.

<hr>

❦

Practical Exercise

If you have not yet worked through chapters 10, 11 and 12, you should do so now, so that you have a good set of coping skills to help you confront your fears about your obsessional thoughts and to cope with your anxiety when you prevent your compulsive behaviors. If you have been using drugs, prescribed or otherwise, to cope with your obsessive-compulsive problem, we strongly encourage you to work through chapter 3 now.

In the space below, try to pinpoint the obsessional thoughts you need to confront. Using chapter 6 as a guide, draw up your plan for doing this. Can you build in a gradual approach?

Obsessional thoughts:

_____

_____

_____

_____

_____

My plan for confronting my obsessional thoughts:

_____

_____

_____

_____

_____

_____

Step 1: _____

Step 2: _____

Step 3: _____

Step 4: _____

Step 5: _____

Step 6: _____

Step 7: _____

Step 8: _____

Step 9: _____

Step 10: _____

Now, in the space below, pinpoint the compulsive behaviors you need to prevent and then create your plan for doing this. Will you need help? Ask your assistants to read the same chapters you have and explain to them exactly how they should help you.

Compulsive behaviors:

_____

_____

_____

_____

(continues)

_____

My plan for preventing my compulsive behaviors:

_____

_____

_____

_____

_____

Step 1: _____

Step 2: _____

Step 3: _____

Step 4: _____

Step 5: _____

Step 6: _____

Step 7: _____

Step 8: _____

Step 9: _____

Step 10: _____

Do you need to prevent compulsive thoughts? Can you distinguish your compulsive thoughts, which you need to prevent, and your obsessive thoughts, which you need to confront? In the space below, brainstorm all of your compulsive and obsessive thoughts. Then put an "O" next to those that cause you anxiety. These are the obsessive thoughts you need to confront. The other thoughts are likely to be the compulsive thoughts you need to prevent. What is your plan for preventing these thoughts? Thought-stopping? Scheduling?

List of obsessive and compulsive thoughts:

_____

_____

_____

_____

_____

_____

_____

_____

My plan for preventing compulsive thoughts:

_____

_____

(continues)

Step 1: _____

Step 2: _____

Step 3: _____

Step 4: _____

Step 5: _____

Step 6: _____

Step 7: _____

Step 8: _____

Step 9: _____

Step 10: _____

Have you developed some habitual rituals that you need to prevent? Remember, a habitual ritual is one that is no longer connected to the anxiety that may have originally started the behavior (see page 135). What is your plan for preventing and eliminating these rituals?

List of habitual rituals:

_____

_____

_____

_____

_____

My plan for preventing and eliminating these rituals:

Step 1: _____

Step 2: _____

Step 3: _____

Step 4: _____

Step 5: _____

Step 6: _____

Step 7: _____

Step 8: _____

Step 9: _____

Step 10: _____

10

How to Manage Anxious Feelings

- Anxiety is an unpleasant state that includes negative feelings, negative thoughts, unpleasant biological reactions and unhelpful shifts in your attention.
- To manage your negative feelings, you will say a coping statement to yourself whenever you feel anxious.
- It also helps you to change your expectations from helplessness toward coping, and to shift your attention away from your anxiety and back to the task at hand.
- The coping statement is a powerful anxiety-management technique, but you will need to use it persistently.

As we discuss in earlier chapters, anxiety is an unpleasant state that includes

- negative emotions (for example, feeling fearful, nervous, jittery, distressed, upset)

145

- expectation of unpleasant or threatening events, inside or outside yourself, but seeing them as unpredictable and out of your control
- shifts in your attention to focus unhelpfully on the possible threats and your reactions to them

You will notice that anxiety is much more than just feelings, although the bad feelings are an important part of it. It also includes thoughts, biological reactions and shifts in your attention. In turn it can prompt behavior, often avoidance of some kind, that eventually makes the problem worse, even if it helps you to avoid feeling anxious in the short term. So we will introduce you to coping skills to manage each of these parts of anxiety. In this chapter, we will introduce a technique for managing anxious feelings. This technique will help you to stop shifting your attention onto your anxiety and to shift it back to the task at hand instead—and it will prompt you to act constructively. The magic wand that does all this is called a *coping statement*.

EXPECTING TO COPE INSTEAD OF COLLAPSE

In chapter 1 we describe how a major part of feeling anxious is believing that you lack control over the situation. You might believe that you will not be able to prevent the expected threat; for example, someone with an obsessive fear of contamination might believe that she won't be able to stop germs from attacking her family. You might believe that you won't be able to react effectively to it when it comes; for example, someone with a social phobia expects to make a fool of himself

This technique will help you to stop shifting your attention onto your anxiety and to shift it back to the task at hand instead—and it will prompt you to act constructively.

when he has to give a speech. You might believe that you won't be able to control your reactions when it comes; for example, someone with a panic problem expects to have an uncontrollable panic attack if she goes to a shopping center.

You will notice that the basic belief in all of these fears is expecting to be helpless, to be overwhelmed by your expected threat or by your reactions to it. We suggest you begin to replace that expectation of helplessness with the more helpful and realistic expectation that you will cope. To do this, you are going to say a coping statement to yourself whenever you feel anxious. Following is the basic formula for a coping statement:

> I expect to feel some anxiety in this situation, but I'll cope; I won't try to deny or avoid my anxiety, but I also won't focus on it or dwell on the problem. If it is possible to do something constructive about the problem now, I'll focus on doing that. If not, I'll focus on doing something else, pleasant or constructive.

Saying a coping statement to yourself should achieve two things:

1. It makes you replace the thoughts that were in your mind with the coping statement. That should help to reduce your anxiety because, as we will show you in chapter 11, the thoughts you were having were most likely increasing your anxiety.
2. The coping statement is a plan for action. It is a set of instructions you give to yourself, whenever you feel anxious. If you act on those instructions as you say them, your anxiety should lessen.

We find people get the best results if they stick closely to our formula, so we encourage you to do the same. To begin, we suggest you write out the coping statement, as it is above, and carry it around with you. The times you will need it most are when you are feeling most anxious and that's when it can be hard to think straight or remember something. If you have the coping statement written on a reminder card, you can pull it out and read it on the spot.

Eventually you will find you have learned it by heart, but there is no need to wait for that.

When you are saying the coping statement, it is important that it means something to you. You will build up your own convictions about its helpfulness as you use it successfully. Let us now give you a head start on that by explaining just how carefully it is designed to give you control over your anxiety.

I EXPECT TO FEEL SOME ANXIETY IN THIS SITUATION

We emphasize again that anxiety is normal in humans. In moderate doses, as a prompt to you to constructively prepare for a possible problem, it can be adaptive. Having some anxious feelings makes you human. You might be able to accept that (and we hope you do), but you might want to insist that your anxiety is "abnormal" because it is excessive or it occurs when there is no real threat. We emphasize that even then you must accept that there is a plausible explanation for why you feel that anxiety.

> To have excessive or inappropriate anxiety is unpleasant and inconvenient, but it's still human.

In the preceding chapters we have outlined what current research tells us about how people probably develop anxiety problems. One of those explanations probably fits you. To have excessive or inappropriate anxiety is unpleasant and inconvenient, but it's still human. Your version of this part of the coping statement might become

I expect to feel anxious in this situation because I have practiced that so much it's going to keep happening for a while . . .

Notice that you are not telling yourself that you are stuck with excessive or inappropriate anxiety, just expecting to keep having some while you work on your program.

It can also help if you fit the coping statement more to yourself, by putting in some details of your anxiety-provoking situation. For example, someone with a general anxiety problem might say, "I expect to feel some anxiety when I worry about what is going to happen tomorrow . . ." Someone with a panic problem, making himself confront the problem, might say, "I expect to feel some anxiety when I go out by myself . . ." Someone with a phobia, making herself confront her unreasonable fears, might say, "I expect to feel some anxiety when there is a loud storm . . ." Someone with a social phobia, making himself confront his unreasonable fear, might say, "I expect to feel some anxiety when I speak to this group . . ." Someone with posttraumatic stress disorder, making herself confront her unreasonable fears, might say, "I expect to feel anxious when I remember what happened to me . . ." Someone with an obsessive-compulsive problem, making herself confront her problem, might say, "I expect to feel some anxiety when I think about the risk of germs infecting my family, but I will stop myself from washing unnecessarily . . . "

In what situations will you be confronting your anxiety?

BUT I'LL COPE

We have emphasized that one of the goals of the coping statement is to shift your reaction to anxiety away from expecting to be helpless to expecting to cope, with the problem or your reactions or both. Not surprisingly, some people have trouble accepting this at first. Partly that's because they have had such a hard time with their anxiety problem that it's now hard for them to feel hopeful. The answer to this is to persist with all of your anxiety-management program, including the coping statement, until you see yourself making progress. Then it becomes easier to believe that you will be able to cope.

> Some people mistakenly think that "to cope" means "to stop feeling anxious."

People's doubts about coping can also result from a mistaken idea about what "cope" means. Some people mistakenly think that "to cope" means "to stop feeling anxious." Since they don't stop feeling anxious, they think they can't be coping. That's wrong. To have no anxiety in a situation actually means you have mastery of that situation: "This truly doesn't affect me at all."

If you persist with your anxiety-management program, you might eventually achieve mastery of a situation that has previously made you feel anxious, although that depends partly on the situation. You might reasonably expect not to feel anxious about writing your name in front of someone else, but most people feel some anxiety about giving a speech to a large audience.

In any case, mastery is not your goal right now. By "cope," we mean "manage" or "get by," and it's important that that's what you mean when you tell yourself you "will cope."

> I expect to have some anxiety in this situation, but I will cope, meaning I will manage my anxiety so that it's no more than it has to be and I will manage the situation constructively.

I WON'T TRY TO DENY OR AVOID MY ANXIETY

Our culture encourages people to deny bad feelings of all kinds, more so for males but also for females. Even when a woman is allowed to show bad feelings more openly, that in turn is often seen as evidence of women's "greater emotionality" and "lack of logic." Certainly men are often still raised to keep a "stiff upper lip" and to regard showing signs of anxiety or fear as "weakness." The problem with trying to deny anxiety is not only that it doesn't work, but it can actually make you feel worse.

Trying to deny anxious feelings can involve your saying things to yourself such as "This is silly. I shouldn't be feeling anxious now." "It's crazy (or weak or cowardly or stupid) to feel like this. What's wrong with me?" It boils down to telling yourself you should not feel anxious. In extreme cases, it involves not even admitting to yourself how bad you are feeling. We think trying to deny your anxiety really is crazy, because normal people have some anxiety. If you make this common mistake, you risk feeling bad about feeling anxious, because you have told yourself that you shouldn't be feeling anxious.

We realize that sounds silly, but look around you at how often people do it—"What's wrong with me? Why am I getting anxious?"—and they get anxious about getting anxious, angry about being anxious or depressed about being anxious.

Attempting to deny your anxiety instead of managing it only makes you feel worse. To help yourself cope better, you will now tell yourself not to try to deny your anxious feelings.

The other way you might try to deny your anxiety is to avoid the situation that triggers it. As you have read, avoidance is one of the defining characteristics of anxiety problems, whether you are avoiding a phobic situation, avoiding going out by yourself, avoiding remembering a past crisis or avoiding an obsessional thought. You will also have read that a major part of solving your anxiety problem is for you to confront your unreasonable fears. This is necessary so that you can experience your learned anxiety to make it possible for it to fade out of your life. This part of the coping statement is your instruction to yourself to stop avoiding and start confronting those fears.

BUT I WON'T FOCUS ON IT OR DWELL ON THE PROBLEM

A shift in attention plays a big role in anxiety problems. As anxiety builds, your attention shifts away from the task at hand. This task may have been the trigger for your anxiety, such as taking an exam, giving a speech, making love or riding in an elevator. Or it may just happen to be what you were supposed to be doing when your anxiety was triggered by something else, such as an intrusive thought, image or memory or something happening around you. Either way, one of the effects of this attention shift is to interfere with your concentration on the task at hand and so reduce your performance. Of course, performing badly could be exactly what you were anxious about. So your anxiety problem becomes a self-fulfilling prediction.

Instead of focusing on the task in hand, you may focus increasingly narrowly on your anxious feelings, on your biological reactions to anxiety, on the threat you expect may come or on your expectations of not handling it effectively or of being overwhelmed by your anxiety. It's not hard to see that the more you focus on any of these, the more anxious you will make yourself. This negative feedback loop is a common part of anxiety problems and explains how your anxiety can keep growing, by feeding on itself.

So that you can perform the task at hand reasonably well and so that you are not letting your anxiety feed on itself, you are now going to instruct yourself to shift your attention away from your anxiety or fears, back to the task you should be concentrating on. And do it! Focus on what you are writing on the exam paper. Concentrate on your speech notes. Pay attention to the nice feelings coming from your lovemaking. Whatever the task is, focus on it.

We realize that this may be difficult for you, especially at first. You might need to consciously and deliberately switch your attention back to the task at hand each time it strays back onto your anxiety, particularly if your anxiety problem is an entrenched habit. But persistence pays off, and the rest of the coping statement is designed to help you.

IF IT IS POSSIBLE TO DO SOMETHING CONSTRUCTIVE ABOUT THE PROBLEM NOW, I'LL FOCUS ON DOING THAT

Anxiety can be adaptive. Feeling anxious about a possible problem can motivate you to do something constructive about it. So it's time for some reality testing. Is the threat that is making you anxious something you can take constructive steps about now? Should you be studying for your exam? Should you be writing notes for your speech or rehearsing it? Will it help you handle your anxiety-provoking situation if you learn to manage your anxious thoughts (see chapter 11), or your physical anxiety (see chapter 12), or if you strengthen your social skills, your sexual skills (see chapter 13) or your interpersonal skills (see chapter 14)?

Sometimes you will be able to take immediate constructive steps to tackle your anxiety problem. But sometimes there won't be steps you can take right away.

IF NOT, I'LL FOCUS ON DOING SOMETHING ELSE, PLEASANT OR CONSTRUCTIVE

Even if the threat that is triggering your anxiety is one you can do something constructive about, you can't and would not want to work on it all the time. There's more to life than preparing for an exam or a speech or strengthening your coping skills. Or there should be! Sometimes when you say the previous part of the coping statement to yourself—"If it is possible to do something constructive about the problem now, I'll focus on doing that"—the answer you will give yourself will be, "Well, there is nothing I can do about that problem right now," or "Well, I have done enough work on that problem for now." In both cases, it's time to do something else.

In some cases, you can't do anything constructive because your anxiety-provoking fears are simply unreasonable. If your anxiety problem involves such unreasonable fears, you will be aware that they are unreasonable. In the next chapter we will give you suggestions on how you attack those unreasonable fears head on, so that they lose their ability to make you anxious. Right now, we want you to stop rehearsing them and increasing your anxiety. Since they are unreasonable, there is nothing to do to prepare for them so, once again, it's time to do something else right now.

You may already have a task or activity you need to concentrate on that your anxiety has distracted you from. Then it's time to make a deliberate effort to shift your attention back onto it. If necessary, keep shifting your attention back to it whenever it strays.

If you don't already have an activity that you should be focusing on, then you need a distraction. You can distract yourself with any activity that will occupy your mind. It could be a constructive, purposeful activity, such as continuing some job or working on a hobby project, or it could be a pleasant activity, such as reading a book, watching a movie, socializing with a friend or some other way of having fun. What matters is that it occupies your mind and holds your attention, so that you aren't tempted to slip back into focusing on your anxiety.

We are talking about aiming for a balance between having some thoughts about possible problems without trying to either deny or exaggerate them. If you bury yourself so completely in distracting activities that you never think about possible threats and never have the chance to experience the normal anxiety associated with them, that becomes avoidance. This is what happens when people develop compulsive behaviors to counter obsessional thoughts. You will not fall into this trap if you follow the coping statement as we have outlined it, because you will first tell yourself to expect some anxiety from your problem and then prompt yourself to find a distracting activity, to prevent an unnecessary increase in your anxiety, not to deny it altogether.

If you find you often need to use this distraction strategy, and many people do when tackling unreasonable fears, it pays to do some planning *before* you need it. If you wait until you are feeling extremely anxious, then conclude that there is nothing you can do about your fears (because they are unreasonable) so you now need a distracting activity, you are not in the best frame of mind for finding one. Use some of the time when you are not feeling so bad to prepare a couple of possible distractions for the rougher times. Get an appealing book or videotape, start a project, line up a friend to visit. Have one or two possible distracting activities ready to go so that the next time you feel bad, it will take little effort to get into one.

A difficult situation for many people is when they have something that needs to be done—a part of their work, a regular

> If you bury yourself so completely in distracting activities that you never think about possible threats and never have the chance to experience the normal anxiety associated with them, that becomes avoidance.

chore—that does not occupy their minds. It's too simple, habitual and routine to need much thought. But it needs to be done and can't easily be postponed until you're in a better frame of mind. So you find yourself mechanically working your way through this activity while your unoccupied mind stews things over, building up your anxiety. In this case you need to find a distracting activity that you can introduce to the situation, one that will not prevent you from completing the necessary tasks but will occupy your spare mental space to prevent any stewing. A lot of people find that something to listen to is helpful, such as a radio program (or even a television program, if the visual distraction won't interfere too much) or an audiocassette or CD. Many cities have audiobook rental stores where you can rent fiction or nonfiction titles just as you'd rent a movie from a video store.

Practical Exercise

Write out several coping statements, each on its own index card, putting in details of your anxiety-provoking situations so that the coping statements apply directly to you. Practice saying the statements to yourself and try to remember to use them whenever you feel anxious. Try to do each of the parts as you say it to yourself. Are there constructive steps you can take to tackle your anxiety-provoking problems? Do you need help with these? Do you need some distracting activities? What will they be? In the space below, brainstorm distracting activities for different situations: at work, at home, in the car, waiting in line, and so forth.

_____

_____

_____

(continues)

11

How to Manage Anxious Thoughts

- Negative thoughts—expecting unpleasant or threatening things to happen, but seeing them as unpredictable and out of control—play a major role in anxiety.
- To prevent negative thoughts from giving you unnecessary anxiety, we suggest you try thinking straight by 1) identifying your anxious thoughts; 2) testing them instead of accepting them; and 3) replacing them with more helpful thoughts.
- It takes persistent practice to change entrenched negative thinking habits.

We have defined anxiety as an unpleasant state that includes negative thoughts. In fact, as we've mentioned, it is our human capacity to think that makes us uniquely vulnerable to anxiety. Certainly, negative thoughts are a major part of anxiety problems. These include expecting unpleasant or threatening things to happen. But you aren't sure when or even if they will happen, even though you expect them. This uncertainty then increases your anxiety.

The unpleasant things might be outside you, such as worrying about the problems you might face today (in general anxiety), worrying about a coming exam (in a social phobia), worrying about getting seriously ill (in a simple phobia), or worrying about being contaminated by dirt (in an obsessive-compulsive problem). Or the unpleasant things might be inside you, such as worrying about having another panic attack (in a panic or agoraphobia problem) or worrying about being overwhelmed by bad feelings if you remember your past crisis experience (in a posttraumatic stress disorder).

A major theme in anxious thoughts is the idea that things are out of your control. These might be the problems or threats that you are expecting. Although you expect them, you probably also see them as unpredictable, which increases your sense of their being out of control. You might believe that, when the threat does occur, you will not be able to act effectively. So again, it is out of your control. Or you may believe that, when the threat does occur, you won't be able to control your anxious reactions to it. Feeling out of control further increases your anxiety. Regaining your sense of being reasonably in control is an important part of solving anxiety problems. Using the coping statement from the previous chapter should help with this. So will challenging and replacing your anxious thoughts, as we will explain below.

In simple terms, the *way* we feel about anything is strongly influenced by *how* we think about it.

There is another important way your thoughts are involved in anxiety, because anxiety also includes unpleasant, negative feelings. As we explain in chapter 1, your thoughts play an important role in all of your feelings, including those you have when you are anxious. In simple terms, the *way* we feel about anything is strongly influenced by *how* we think about it. If you have bad feelings that are so strong or long-lasting that they are interfering with your life, chances are that you are unnecessarily adding to your bad feelings by how you are thinking. In this chapter we will show you how to stop doing that.

FEELING BETTER BY THINKING STRAIGHTER

The key idea behind this technique is to stop just accepting your thoughts automatically as if they were true and instead to question them. This involves looking for evidence for and against your original thoughts, looking for alternative explanations for the situation, identifying more realistic possible outcomes than the ones you are getting anxious about, coming up with more helpful thoughts, pushing yourself into constructive action, and getting some perspective on your problem. If that seems a mouthful, don't worry, because you will take it one step at a time and we'll give you lots of examples to guide your own efforts. Those steps are set out on page 175 in the exercise, Questioning Your Thoughts: Feeling Better and Acting Constructively. We suggest you don't write on that page but use it to make copies for your own use. Photocopies are great, but you can write the headings on any blank sheet of paper. We do find that people master this skill better if they write it out for a while. If you are seeing a psychologist or other counselor, your written exercises will be good for the two of you to review together. Now, let's show you how to question your thoughts and act constructively.

AN EXAMPLE OF QUESTIONING YOUR THOUGHTS IN GENERAL ANXIETY

In this first example, we'll explain each step as we go. Sample responses follow each step.

Briefly describe the problem: Write a brief description of the situation making you anxious: what is happening, where, when, who is doing what.

> Home during the day, I'm worrying about my husband and kids; are they OK? Has anything bad happened to them? Will my husband have a good day at work? Will the kids get home from school OK? What if one of them catches the flu that's going around? Won't we all get it then? Ring my husband at work twice, even though he obviously thinks I'm being silly. Think I'll drive down and pick up the kids after

school, even though it's close and they prefer to walk home with their friends. I really start to worry if anyone's late home.

And how it makes you feel: Briefly describe your feelings, your emotions, *not* your thoughts.

Edgy and tense, restless and shaky; if I worry a lot, I start to feel sick.

And what you think about it: What are the thoughts in your mind relevant to the problem? Humans do lots of thinking in images rather than words, but you can still describe those images.

I'm imagining my husband having more problems at work and coming home upset, and that upsetting the whole family. I'm imagining something bad happening to the kids, like a road accident on the way home, and one or both of them being hurt or even killed.

What is the evidence that *supports* your thoughts? There will usually be some evidence, because your thoughts are usually not totally impossible, just very exaggerated.

My husband does have bad days at work now and then, and it does upset all of us if he's upset. Accidents do sometimes happen to children on the street. They are a bit later getting home than usual now.

What is the evidence *against* your thoughts? There will always be some evidence, because your anxious thoughts are exaggerated, and you may be ignoring some obvious contradictory evidence.

Most days his work is fine, and he is too; even sometimes when he does come home upset, we can cheer him up as a family. If anything did happen to the kids at school, the school would contact me. There hasn't been an accident involving children on our street ever, and our kids are sensible.

Is there an alternative explanation for what happened? Other than the dreadful one you cooked up? Something less worrying and more likely?

There is no good reason for me to be concerned; it's my unnecessary worrying that's making me feel bad, not any real problem. There are plenty of good reasons why one of the family might be a bit late, without my imagining bad ones.

What is the worst that could happen? What is the absolutely, extremely worst outcome, even if it's unlikely or nearly impossible?

He would have a bad day at work, come home unhappy, and we'd have an unpleasant evening. Something could go wrong with one or both of the kids.

Could you live through it? Not, would you want this outcome, but, if it actually happened, could you cope with that?

Yes; I'd rather not, but if I had to, I could cope with it.

What is the best that could happen? What is the absolutely, extremely best outcome, even if it's unlikely or nearly impossible?

Nothing bad ever happens to any of us, and I don't worry unnecessarily ever again.

What is the most realistic outcome? This will usually be somewhere in between the two extremes you have just cooked up above.

We will occasionally have our share of bad luck, but we'll cope with that. I can gradually reduce my unnecessary worrying and stop myself from doing worry behaviors.

What is the effect of believing your original thoughts about this? How you feel depends a lot on how you think; how does thinking and believing your original thoughts make you feel?

The more I believe my worrying, the more tense, edgy, restless, shaky and nervous I feel.

What could be the effect of questioning those thoughts? If you can question your original thoughts working through this exercise, how does that change your feelings?

> I feel less bad, and I'm less pushed to do my worry behaviors.

What should you do about this problem? You're thinking straighter now, so back that up with some constructive action on the problem if you can, or occupy your mind with something if you can't get at this problem now.

> We can take the usual precautions that any reasonable family might take, but that's as much as I should do. When I catch myself starting to worry unnecessarily, make myself say a coping statement (from chapter 10) instead, and then focus on a pleasant or constructive activity, but don't do any worry behavior. If that makes me tense, I can use my relaxation skills (from chapter 12). I can also do a QYT exercise (from chapter 11) to challenge my worrying thoughts.

What would you say to a friend if s/he were in the same situation? Detaching from a problem helps you to see it in perspective; if this was your friend's problem, not yours, what advice would you give your friend?

> Excessive worrying never stopped anything bad from happening; it just makes you feel anxious (believe me, I know). Take reasonable precautions, then occupy your mind with something more useful than worrying

Well done!

AN EXAMPLE OF QUESTIONING YOUR THOUGHTS FOR PANIC AND AGORAPHOBIA

This time, we'll do the example as you might, without any explanation from us. If you're not sure what a step is about, go back and read the same step in the previous example.

Briefly describe the problem:

Ever since I had a panic attack at the shopping mall, I haven't been able to go there without my mother. If I try to, I start to have another panic attack and have to come home. Mom doesn't mind going with me, but I want to be able to do it by myself again, like I used to. I hate having this problem.

And how it makes you feel:

My heart races, I perspire even when it's cold, I feel dizzy and strange like I'm going to collapse, and I'm frightened I'll have another panic attack and they'll take me to the hospital again. I'm depressed about how this has affected my life.

And what you think about it:

If I go to the mall alone, I'll have another panic attack. If my heart starts to beat faster, it means I'm going to have another panic attack. I'm weak for being like this; I'm never going to be normal again.

What is the evidence that *supports* your thoughts?

I did have a panic attack in the mall before, and it did start with my heart racing. No one else I know has this problem, and I haven't been able to get rid of it.

What is the evidence *against* your thoughts?

I didn't have panic attacks before, and I used to be fine going out by myself; I don't have a panic attack every time my heart speeds up. Plenty of other people have had panic problems and solved them successfully.

Is there an alternative explanation for what happened?

Now I can see the factors that triggered my first panic attack: being hot, hassled by the crowds, worried about the kids, then overreacting to my physical responses. My heart rate will vary all the time, like everyone's, but it doesn't mean I have to have a panic attack.

What is the worst that could happen?

I have another panic attack when I go to the mall by myself or whenever my heart rate increases. So I never go out by myself again.

Could you live through it?

Don't want to, but I could cope if I had to.

What is the best that could happen?

I would never have a panic attack again in my life, and I would immediately feel completely comfortable going out by myself.

What is the most realistic outcome?

I will gradually prove to myself that I can go out alone again and I can put the brakes on my physical anxiety reactions when I need to. Eventually, I won't be seriously troubled by feelings of panic.

What is the effect of believing your original thoughts about this?

I worry about going out alone so much that I avoid it; I overreact when I get any physical signs of anxiety—I panic about having a panic attack.

What could be the effect of questioning those thoughts?

I feel less worried about going out alone and less anxious when I notice my heart beating, so I'm less likely to have another panic attack.

What should you do about this problem?

Practice the coping statement (from chapter 10) and my calming response (from chapter 12) to use when I start to get physical signs of anxiety; and then draw up and stick to my plan (from chapter 6) for confronting my fears about going out alone.

What would you say to a friend if s/he were in the same situation?

I can see this has become a bad problem for you and that must be distressing, but you have a constructive plan for solving it now. Go to it and take it a step at a time.

AN EXAMPLE OF QUESTIONING YOUR THOUGHTS FOR A PHOBIA

Briefly describe the problem:

Whenever I try to ride in an elevator, I feel so anxious that I think I'm going to be sick. I just can't ride in them, and sometimes that's a real nuisance.

And how it makes you feel:

Really frightened and then nauseous; a bit embarrassed if I think someone notices me trying to go in and then walking away.

And what you think about it:

If I get in the elevator, I'll get so frightened that I will be sick and I won't be able to get out until it stops at a floor. If there's anyone else there, they'll think I'm crazy.

What is the evidence that *supports* your thoughts?

I do feel frightened about riding in elevators at present, and it's true you can't get out until it stops and the doors open. I have heard about some accidents involving elevators.

What is the evidence *against* your thoughts?

Riding in an elevator is definitely safer than riding in a car. I can do lots of other riskier things without being too frightened. I had to overcome my fears for some of those too, and I did.

Is there an alternative explanation for what happened?

Somewhere I have learned to be frightened of riding in elevators, and it's only natural that being in a situation where I can't easily escape adds to my anxiety.

What is the worst that could happen?

I push myself to ride an elevator and get very frightened, maybe even nauseous, and maybe someone else does think I'm strange.

Could you live through it?

Yes, none of that's the end of the world.

What is the best that could happen?

I would never feel anxious about riding in an elevator again in my life.

What is the most realistic outcome?

I will gradually prove to myself that I can ride in an elevator and I can put the brakes on any anxiety reactions when I need to.

What is the effect of believing your original thoughts about this?

I get too anxious to use an elevator, even when it would save me a lot of walking. It's very inconvenient, but I also feel silly about it.

What could be the effect of questioning those thoughts?

I feel less worried about riding in an elevator and feeling anxious when I do.

What should you do about this problem?

Practice the coping statement (from chapter 10) and my calming response (from chapter 12) to use when I start to feel anxious; and then draw up and stick to my plan (from chapter 6) for confronting my fears about riding in elevators.

What would you say to a friend if s/he were in the same situation?

This isn't worth the wear and tear on your feet; you have a plan for overcoming your fear of elevators. Go to it and take it one step at a time.

AN EXAMPLE OF QUESTIONING YOUR THOUGHTS FOR A SOCIAL PHOBIA

Briefly describe the problem:

I have to give a sales report to a management meeting every week at work, and I'm finding it increasingly difficult. I get really tense, and then I rush to get it over. Sometimes, because I'm rushing and uptight, I lose my thread and make a mess of it.

And how it makes you feel:

Anxious, tense, flustered, and embarrassed when I notice how badly I'm doing.

And what you think about it:

Everyone else does their presentations fine; I'm the only one who always makes a mess of it. The boss must think I'm hopeless.

What is the evidence that *supports* your thoughts?

I do tend to rush my presentations, sometimes lose my thread, and so I'm not doing them as well as I want to. I probably don't make as good an impression as I would like to.

What is the evidence *against* your thoughts?

No one, including the boss, has been very critical of my presentations. In fact, they usually pay close attention.

Is there an alternative explanation for what happened?

I have learned to worry so much about how other people judge my performance that I make myself anxious and don't do as well as I could. But I learned to do all that, I'm not stuck with it.

What is the worst that could happen?

I not only never get any better, but I actually get worse and never get promoted, maybe I'll get fired. They all think I'm an idiot.

Could you live through it?

Don't want to, but I could cope if I had to.

What is the best that could happen?

I would immediately feel completely comfortable doing my presentations and so always do them excellently without ever making a mistake. They all decide I am perfect and I keep getting promotions.

What is the most realistic outcome?

I will gradually feel less anxious about making presentations and so my performance will gradually get better by not being hindered by my anxiety. I'll get reasonable approval from my boss and my colleagues.

What is the effect of believing your original thoughts about this?

I worry about doing a bad presentation so much that I don't do a good one. A couple of times I've tried to get out of it, which would not really be good for my reputation.

What could be the effect of questioning those thoughts?

I feel less anxious before and during my presentation, so I can focus on it better and go at a better pace.

What should you do about this problem?

Practice the coping statement (from chapter 10) before a presentation, and use the calming response (from chapter 12) during a presentation if I feel anxious; make sure I have put in reasonable preparation for each presentation and check out whether there are any skills or extra training I would benefit from for my job or presentations.

What would you say to a friend if s/he were in the same situation?

From the reactions of the other people in the situation, you seem to already be doing OK, but I'm sure you can improve if you work systematically on your anxiety.

AN EXAMPLE OF STRAIGHT THINKING FOR POSTTRAUMATIC STRESS

Briefly describe the problem:

Ever since my car accident, I just can't ride in a car unless I'm driving, and even then I don't want to go on roads where the traffic is fast. I've been staying away from my lawn bowls club in case anyone asks me about the accident, because I just don't want to talk about it; it brings back such bad memories.

And how it makes you feel:

Very panicky and out of control.

And what you think about it:

Anything that reminds me of the accident makes it flash through my mind again, and I feel so bad I don't think I can control my reactions.

What is the evidence that *supports* your thoughts?

It was a bad accident and a terrifying experience. Whenever I have allowed myself to remember it, I have been very distressed.

What is the evidence *against* your thoughts?

If I have avoided being reminded about the accident, then I can't really know how I would cope with the memories if I stopped avoiding them.

Is there an alternative explanation for what happened?

My reactions at the time of the accident and afterwards are just how everybody reacts in similar circumstances, including my trying to avoid reminders. But that's what has stopped me from proving to myself that I can cope with those bad memories; I've never really given myself the chance to.

What is the worst that could happen?

If I let myself be reminded of my accident, I might feel very bad, maybe nearly as bad as I did then, and maybe I won't be able to control my emotions for a while.

Could you live through it?

Don't want to, but I could cope if I had to.

What is the best that could happen?

I could be reminded of my accident, talk about it in detail to anyone, and never feel any discomfort ever again.

What is the most realistic outcome?

I will gradually prove to myself that I can be reminded of my accident and I can put the brakes on my unpleasant reactions when I need to. Eventually I won't be seriously troubled by memories of my accident; I'll get it into perspective as an ugly memory when I'm reminded of it, but not one that dominates or interferes with my life.

What is the effect of believing your original thoughts about this?

I feel frightened that I'm going to be overwhelmed by bad memories and my emotional reactions to them, so frightened that I've been avoiding any reminders, and this is restricting my life.

What could be the effect of questioning those thoughts?

I could feel less anxious about reminders, and so have less need to avoid them; I could rebuild my life.

What should you do about this problem?

Practice the coping statement (from chapter 10) and my calming response (from chapter 12) to use when I allow myself to be reminded of my accident; and then draw up and stick to my plan (from chapter 6) for confronting my fears about being reminded.

What would you say to a friend if s/he were in the same situation?

The accident was very bad, and it makes sense that it has upset you so badly, but now you are letting it interfere in your life more than it needs to. You have a constructive plan for overcoming it now. Take it a step at a time.

AN EXAMPLE OF STRAIGHT THINKING FOR AN OBSESSIVE-COMPULSIVE PROBLEM

Briefly describe the problem:

I keep thinking that my hands are dirty, especially but not only when I've been working in the garden, and that I'm going to spread germs inside the house and make the whole family sick. So I keep washing my hands, lots of times every day. That makes me feel relieved for a little while. But then it all happens again. I know this is ridiculous, but I just can't stop.

And how it makes you feel:

Anxious and worried until I wash my hands, and even then I feel silly because I know it was unnecessary. I'm getting really depressed about being stuck like this and the problems it's causing the rest of the family.

And what you think about it:

There are germs everywhere, especially wherever it's dirty. If I don't wash them off properly, they'll make someone in the family sick, maybe they'll die. I know I'm over the top about this, but I can't help it.

What is the evidence that *supports* your thoughts?

There are germs in the world, and some of them can make people sick. But none of my friends takes hygiene to such a ridiculous level.

What is the evidence *against* your thoughts?

Most germs are harmless or even helpful to humans. People who set reasonable standards of hygiene don't get sick from a lack of cleanliness.

Is there an alternative explanation for what happened?

Somehow I have learned an exaggerated fear of germs and illness, and I have learned the bad habit of excessive washing to cope with the anxiety caused by my exaggerated fear. Like other anxiety problems, it keeps itself going.

What is the worst that could happen?

I fail to keep reasonable hygiene, and someone does actually get sick because of it.

Could you live through it?

Don't want to, but I could cope if I had to.

What is the best that could happen?

I would immediately stop having exaggerated fears of germs and sickness and would always comfortably be able to stick to reasonable standards of cleanliness.

What is the most realistic outcome?

I will gradually prove to myself that I can stick to reasonable standards of cleanliness and I can put the brakes on my anxious reactions when I stop myself, preferably with some help, from excessive washing.

What is the effect of believing your original thoughts about this?

I worry so much about germs and illness that I wash my hands much more than I really need to. I'm hurting the skin on my hands, upsetting my family and myself.

What could be the effect of questioning those thoughts?

I feel less worried about germs and sickness and able to begin stopping my unnecessary washing and eventually able to set reasonable hygiene limits.

What should you do about this problem?

Practice the coping statement (from chapter 10) and my calming response (from chapter 12) to use when I begin to stop all unreasonable washing (as explained in chapter 9); and then draw up and stick to my plan for doing this, preferably with some help.

What would you say to a friend if s/he were in the same situation?

Of course you're going to feel bad about this, because it looks so strange. But you did learn it; so have plenty of other people, and they have solved their problems. You have a constructive plan for solving it now. Get some help and take it one step at a time.

YOUR TURN

OK, that's enough examples. We hope that one or two of them are similar to your anxiety problem, but even if they're not, the principles apply to everybody. In fact, questioning your thoughts is a really useful life skill that you can get benefit from, long after you have solved your anxiety problem. We find it's helpful for people trying to manage depression or cope with stress or tackle just about any problem. We encourage you to take some time now to get good at it. Make your own copies of the QYT form, or transfer the headings to some blank pages and try some straight thinking for your anxiety problem. And back it up with some constructive action. Not sure what to do? You may well find some of the action answers you're looking for in chapters 13 and 14, but spend some time on your straight thinking practice.

❧

Questioning Your Thoughts: Feeling Better and Acting Constructively

Briefly describe the problem:

_____

_____

_____

_____

And how it makes you feel:

_____

_____

_____

_____

And what you think about it:

_____

_____

_____

_____

(continues)

What is the evidence that *supports* your thoughts?

_____

_____

_____

_____

What is the evidence *against* your thoughts?

_____

_____

_____

_____

Is there an alternative explanation for what happened?

_____

_____

_____

_____

What is the worst that could happen?

_____

_____

_____

_____

Could you live through it?

_____

_____

_____

_____

What is the best that could happen?

_____

_____

_____

_____

What is the most realistic outcome?

_____

_____

_____

_____

What is the effect of believing your original thoughts about this?

_____

_____

_____

_____

(continues)

What could be the effect of questioning those thoughts?

_____

_____

_____

_____

What should you do about this problem?

_____

_____

_____

_____

What would you say to a friend if s/he were in the same situation?

_____

_____

_____

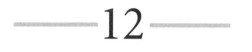

12

How to Manage Physical Anxiety

- Anxiety includes a number of physical symptoms. Focusing on them can increase your anxiety.
- A coping statement and straight thinking will help you to avoid misinterpreting signs of physical arousal.
- Drugs do not help with and can cause physical anxiety symptoms.
- Regular moderate exercise can help with stress and anxiety.
- You can learn the calming response to relax quickly in anxiety-provoking situations.
- You can learn deep relaxation to counter the tension of physical anxiety and help you sleep.
- Disturbed sleep is a common result of anxiety, although sleeping problems usually involve other factors as well.
- Sleeping drugs make sleeping problems worse.
- To sleep better you need to identify the causes of your sleeping problem and tackle all of them systematically.

Anxiety is an unpleasant state that can include a number of physical symptoms, such as:

- skipping, racing or pounding of the heart (palpitations)
- pain, pressure or tightness in the chest
- tingling or numbness in the toes or fingers
- butterflies or discomfort in the stomach
- constipation or diarrhea
- restlessness or jumpiness
- tight, tense muscles
- sweating not brought on by heat
- a lump in the throat
- trembling or shaking
- rubbery or "jelly" legs
- feeling dizzy, lightheaded or off balance
- choking or smothering sensations or difficulty breathing
- headaches or pains in the neck or back
- hot flushes or cold chills
- feeling tired, weak or easily exhausted

Recognize any of these? At least a few of these physical symptoms will occur with all anxiety problems. They add to the unpleasantness of anxiety, especially if you worry about them. Shifting your attention from the task at hand onto the physical symptoms of your anxiety is a common part of anxiety problems, causing your anxiety to feed on itself. The extreme example of this is what happens with panic and agoraphobia problems, as we explain in chapter five.

> Shifting your attention from the task at hand onto the physical symptoms of your anxiety is a common part of anxiety problems, causing your anxiety to feed on itself.

INTERPRETING PHYSICAL ANXIETY SYMPTOMS

In chapter five we also explain how you can unnecessarily increase your anxiety by misinterpreting signs of increased physical arousal. For example, you may notice your breathing has become faster but, instead of recognizing that that is due to your just walking up the stairs, you tell yourself you are about to feel anxious (again). A very common misinterpretation is to believe that anxiety-produced pain or tightness in your chest signals an impending heart attack. A 1987 research study found that a high proportion of patients going to heart specialists because of chest pain in fact had normal coronary arteries (the ones usually blocked in heart disease) and instead had a panic problem.

We won't encourage you to ignore chest pain, or any other strong physical symptoms, especially not if they are new for you. Take the common sense precaution of having your physical health checked by your doctor. But, when you are told there is nothing physically wrong with you, we suggest you take that advice to heart (no pun intended) and stop misinterpreting any signs of increased physical arousal. You can use the coping skills in the previous two chapters to manage your *reactions* to your physical symptoms, and you can use the coping skills in this chapter to manage the physical symptoms themselves.

PHYSICAL ANXIETY AND MEDICATION

We consider drugs and anxiety at length in chapter three. A couple of points are important to bring up again.

1. Drinking too much caffeine can cause biological arousal and contribute to anxiety.
2. Drinking too much alcohol may give you an overdose of one of its byproducts, lactate, which seems to increase anxiety.

We have mentioned that antianxiety drugs have a poor record for helping with anxiety, especially in the long run, but we repeat here the concern of some medical authorities that antianxiety drugs can *cause* some of the symptoms of anxiety. There is also the strong risk of your becoming dependent on them so that when you try to stop taking an antianxiety drug, you suffer a withdrawal reaction, including unpleasant physical symptoms. We cannot recommend drugs of any kind for managing your physical anxiety.

PHYSICAL ANXIETY AND EXERCISE

In chapter two we discuss how stress leads to anxiety. One of the consequences of too much stress is chronic fatigue, which you will notice is also among the physical symptoms of anxiety listed above. As a part of stress management, we recommend a program of regular, moderate exercise. We emphasize *moderate.* This is exercise for ordinary people, not fitness fanatics. It increases your ability to cope with the life demands that are putting stress on you, reducing your risk of fatigue and therefore helping you to lead a balanced lifestyle. Regular moderate exercise can help you with anxiety management as well. It will help you to avoid unnecessary physical arousal from exertion and to feel more in control of your body's reactions.

LEARN TO RELAX QUICKLY

Anxiety tends to feed on itself. Shifting your attention to your anxious reactions, including your physical reactions, prompts you to feel anxious about how anxious you are becoming. Feeling unable to control your reactions further increases your anxiety. As you may have noticed, this can all happen rapidly, leaving you feeling overwhelmed by your anxiety. So it will be helpful if you can do something just as quickly, on the spot, to slow down your physical reactions and help you regain your sense of being in control of yourself. That's what you will use the calming response for.

This is a quick and brief coping skill, based on the "quieting response" for stress-management developed by Dr. Charles Stroebel and his colleagues. This technique is helpful for people who have a problem with strong reactions that develop quickly, such as anger, but it is also helpful for anxiety, especially for panic problems.

THE CALMING RESPONSE

Step 1   Mentally detach from the situation and smile to yourself.

Step 2   Think, *Clear head, calm body.*

Step 3   Take in one slow, deep breath.

Step 4   As you breathe out, relax your body, from your head to your toes.

The calming response is most effective if you use it early, before your anxiety level is too high. So the first trick is to learn your own early warning signs. What do you notice in your situation or in yourself that warns you that you are about to become anxious? Learn what your early warning signs are and use them to prompt you to start a calming response. The calming response takes only about six seconds, so you can do it on the spot without interfering with the task at hand. Other people will only notice that you are being thoughtful, which won't hurt your image.

Step 1 Mentally detach from the situation and smile to yourself.

As soon as you can step back from the situation, even mentally, it has less impact on you. Smiling to yourself helps that detachment and adds the calming effect of humor. Just make sure you are smiling to yourself and not grinning at everybody else.

Step 2 Think, *Clear head, calm body.*

You are telling yourself that your mind will stay alert while you deal with the situation, preferably focusing on the task at hand, but your body is about to relax.

Step 3 Take in one slow, deep breath.

Fast, shallow or irregular breathing is a common physical symptom of anxiety. Taking control of your breathing, slowing it down, helps you to feel in control of yourself.

Step 4 As you breathe out, relax your body, from your head to your feet.

Imagine a wave of relaxation, starting in your head and flowing down through your body to your feet. Let the tension melt out of your body, like butter in the sun.

The calming response is a practical skill, so you will get better at it with practice. We suggest a couple minutes each day. Lots of little practices work better than occasional long ones. Imagine yourself in an anxiety-provoking situation. Take enough time to make it realistic for you. Imagine your anxious feelings and physical reactions. Then imagine your way through the calming response, one step at a time. Imagine yourself successfully calming down your reactions and regaining your sense of being in control. This rehearsal in your imagination is good preparation for using the calming response in real situations.

Practical Exercise

Read over the instructions for the calming response and make sure you understand them. Write out a short summary of the instructions, so that you can carry it as a reminder while you are learning it. Think of some situations in which it will be helpful to you and jot them down in the space below. Pick some times when you can practice in your imagination. You only need a couple of spare minutes each time. Then start some regular practice, until the calming response has become your habitual way of reacting to an increase in your arousal.

_____

_____

_____

LEARN TO RELAX DEEPLY

Relaxation training is often touted as a magical cure-all, which it definitely is not in and of itself. In fact, if all you learn to do is relax your body, the mere act of trying to do this can actually make you more tense. You may use your "relaxation time" as uncluttered worry time. If intrusive thoughts and worries interfere with your attempts to relax, you will need to deal with them first by working through chapters 10 and 11.

Some people say that they can relax during their relaxation class or while at home or on vacation, but not in their anxiety-provoking situations. In situations where you have a task to complete, deep relaxation may be inappropriate, anyway, because it takes too long. The calming response described above is more appropriate for those times. Some people with anxiety problems experience deep relaxation as a loss of control, which actually increases anxiety. In this case, you are better off directing your attention to a purposeful activity, either the task at hand or some distracting activity (see the coping statement in chapter 10, page 147).

Deep relaxation can be a useful anxiety-management technique, however, when it is part of a total program, such as the one we hope you have planned for yourself by now. So we suggest you learn how to relax deeply and try it for managing your physical anxiety. It can be an effective counter to the symptoms of physical tension and it can help you sleep better, something we address shortly.

You can't easily learn physical relaxation from a book. It's difficult to read and turn the pages while trying to relax deeply. One good way is to go to a relaxation training course, such as those offered by community centers and colleges. Another possibility is a yoga class, although some yoga teachers make exaggerated claims about what they can help people with. Skip the hype and learn to relax, if yoga suits you.

Similar reservations apply to flotation tanks, biofeedback training and other gadgets marketed with quite remarkable claims. Careful research has found that the various relaxation techniques are all about as effective as each other. So we suggest you try a low-cost approach first.

A method that many people have found helpful is to teach yourself to relax while listening to instructions on an audiocassette. You can do it whenever you want, without having to travel to a class, and it's cheaper. Look for a plain, straightforward relaxation training tape on which you can hear clear instructions on what to do. We definitely do not recommend so-called "subliminal suggestion" tapes, not for relaxation or anything else. There is no scientific evidence that these ever helped anybody and there are solid scientific reasons why they never could. Don't waste your money.

If you are willing to do a little work, you can make your own relaxation tape. All you need is a simple cassette recorder, a blank cassette tape, and a script of relaxation instructions. We include a suitable script and some suggestions on how to use it at the end of this chapter.

Careful research has found that the various relaxation techniques are all about as effective as each other. So we suggest you try a low-cost approach first.

Practical Exercise

In the space below, write out your plan for learning to relax deeply. Take a class? Which one? Use a relaxation training cassette? Will you buy one or make one? When will you start? (How about soon?)

_____

_____

_____

_____

_____

SLEEPING BETTER WITHOUT DRUGS

Insomnia, or disturbed sleep, is a common reaction to anxiety. It is often reported by people with general anxiety and other anxiety problems. If you go to bed in a high state of arousal because of your anxiety or use bed as a place to rehearse your worries, it's not surprising that you have trouble sleeping. In children, who may have trouble describing or talking about their anxiety or worries, disturbed sleep may be the most obvious sign of how anxious they are.

Insomnia is not a life-threatening problem, so it is not always taken seriously. If your sleep is disturbed, however, you know just how disruptive it can be. Technically, insomnia is defined as poor sleep accompanied by daytime fatigue. This includes being physically tired, having difficulty concentrating, feeling depressed, irritable or lethargic. These daytime components of insomnia are the problem and, because they interfere with your ability to cope with daytime

> Insomnia is not a life-threatening problem, so it is not always taken seriously. If your sleep is disturbed, however, you know just how disruptive it can be.

tasks, they further increase your stress and therefore your anxiety. In yet another way, anxiety can feed on itself.

WHAT IS SLEEP?

Sleep is more than just not being awake. There are five different levels of sleep, and levels 1 through 4 consist of light to very deep sleep. You normally move back and forth through these levels during sleep, reaching level 4, the deepest, a couple of hours after falling asleep. Level 5 is the strange one because it is marked by activity in the brain similar to that of someone who is awake. The sleeper's eyes move rapidly under her closed eyelids, which is why this level is sometimes called *REM* (rapid eye movement) sleep. Yet her body muscles have reached their deepest level of relaxation. If you wake a sleeper during level 5, she will often report that she was dreaming. Although many of us don't remember much or anything about our dreams, sleep researchers have found that all of their subjects had several periods of REM sleep each night, so dreaming seems to be a normal and nightly occurrence.

We really don't know why humans need to sleep, but there is little doubt about how disruptive a lack of good sleep can be. In particular it seems that we need levels 3, 4 and REM sleep, to function normally during the day. If you are somehow deprived of REM sleep, eventually your body will catch up by having lots of it. However this rebound effect is usually marked by vivid dreams or nightmares and therefore disturbed sleep. We have taken time to explain all of this to you, not because you need to be an instant expert on sleep theory, but because it has important implications for what you do about disturbed sleep.

HOW MUCH SLEEP DO YOU NEED?

Sleep needs vary a lot and tend to decline with increasing age. Although some insomnia sufferers will complain they "didn't get a wink," research has found they usually did sleep for at least a few hours. Complete insomnia is a rare condition. One bad night's sleep, even as little as two hours, doesn't really affect your performance the next day, although you may feel more irritable, hostile, fatigued or unhappy. Little sleep for a week makes some people pathologically sleepy, but even these cumulative effects disappear after one good night's sleep. So the real question is not how much time you spend asleep, but how you feel during the day. If your sleep disturbance is caused by your anxiety problem, you might expect it to fade as you learn to manage your anxiety. This is possible but there is one risk.

For some insomnia sufferers, disturbed sleep was triggered by some easily identifiable cause: a painful illness, jetlag, a peak of stress, whatever. But after the original cause has long faded from the person's life, his sleep is still disturbed because it has become a conditioned part of his life. He has learned that bed is somewhere he vainly tries to sleep and approaching sleep causes anxiety about "another sleepless night." He may also have tried some of the popular remedies for sleeping problems that actually make them worse, or developed some bad sleep habits that now keep his problem going. If you are now having more than the occasional night of disturbed sleep, we suggest you take some practical steps to sleep better to avoid the risk of developing a long-term sleeping problem.

Little sleep for a week makes some people pathologically sleepy, but even these cumulative effects disappear after one good night's sleep.

WHAT DISTURBS YOUR SLEEP?

Sleep researchers agree that insomnia is not an illness but a symptom of underlying problems, just as a pain signifies something else is wrong. There are five groups of factors that contribute to insomnia:

1. biological factors
2. psychological factors
3. use of drugs, including alcohol
4. bad sleep habits or environments
5. conditioning

The specialists in treating sleep disorders agree on two more important points. First, they never see someone with a sleep disturbance due to only one of these possible factors. Significant sleep problems always reflect the interaction of several of these possible causes. Second, they agree that successfully solving a sleep problem requires carefully identifying the causes applying to each person, so that she tackles all of those relevant to her. The point about these conclusions is that even if your anxiety problem clearly contributes to your sleep problem, there are probably other factors involved as well. If you want to solve your sleeping problem now, you need to identify all of its possible causes and do something constructive about them. To help you do some self-diagnosis and plan your personal sleep-management program, we will describe those five possible factors.

Biological factors. Sleep and wakefulness are probably governed by two brain systems: an arousal system and a sleep system. For sleep to occur, the sleep system has to override the arousal system. Psychologist Peter Hauri, who is director of the Sleep Disorders Clinic at Dartmouth Medical School, believes that some insomniacs may have strong arousal systems or weak sleep systems. Compared to sound sleepers, insomniacs do have higher levels of physiological arousal even when they are having a good night's sleep. We have already mentioned the research evidence that suggests that people who develop anxiety problems are vulnerable to this because they have inherited overreactive nervous systems. The implication of this is that your sleep will benefit if you are able to deliver yourself to bed in a physically relaxed state.

Medical problems can also disturb sleep. Potential culprits are arthritis, ulcers, angina, migraines and other physical pain; asthma, sleep apnea (brief periods of not breathing) and other breathing disorders; irregular heartbeat; kidney disease; thyroid gland problems; pregnancy; and jerky spasms in your large muscles (called *nocturnal myoclonus*), especially in the legs. Since these are medical problems, you should be getting medical treatment for them.

The normal, gradual decline in your sleep needs as you get older can cause problems if you start to worry about not getting as much sleep as you used to. You can reassure yourself that, unless it is associated with the daytime consequences of insomnia, sleeping less as you age is not a problem.

Psychological factors. The psychological problem most likely to contribute to insomnia is anxiety, which in turn increases your physiological arousal. Insomnia is a common symptom of high stress and, by interfering with daytime functioning, it can further add to stress. Some depressed people suffer from disturbed or shortened sleep, although some sleep more than usual. That this is still a sleep disturbance is shown by the fact that these people report being fatigued, despite their extra sleep.

Use of drugs. Many drugs, including alcohol, can disturb your sleep. This includes legal and illegal, prescribed, over-the-counter and social drugs. In one research study, drug or alcohol dependency was found to be a major cause of insomnia for one in eight sufferers. Sleep clinicians have found that many types of antianxiety, antidepression and other mood-affecting drugs can disturb sleep. So can some of the drugs used for thyroid problems, contraception and heart disease. If you are taking any regular medication you should ask your doctor whether it could be contributing to your sleeping problem and, if it could, whether you can try a different drug or even a nondrug treatment.

What may surprise you, however, is that sleeping drugs themselves contribute to sleep disturbance. That's right, the drugs recommended to treat your sleeping problem can make it worse. This is obviously important and it may be confusing for you: one "expert" is suggesting you take these drugs while some other "experts" (us) are suggesting you don't. So let us explain our doubts about sleeping drugs so that you can make your own informed decision.

> What may surprise you, however, is that sleeping drugs themselves contribute to sleep disturbance.

Sleeping drugs usually put you to sleep, so they seem to work. The trouble is, they knock out the lower levels of sleep, the ones that are essential for your refreshment. They cause fragmented and disturbed sleep, shortened REM sleep periods and frequent early waking. Because of these unwanted side effects, you may spend time asleep but without getting the benefit of normal sleep. As with antianxiety drugs, your body can become accustomed to the sleeping drug so that you have to keep increasing the dose to get any effect until even taking the maximum safe dose is no longer effective. Many patients have wound up hooked on their sleeping drugs, with a drug dependency problem as well as an unsolved sleeping problem.

Because sleeping drugs reduce your REM sleep periods, if you stop taking the drug you then have the rebound effect we described earlier, with vivid dreams and nightmares. Many people have misinterpreted this rebound sleep disturbance as meaning they needed to stay on their sleeping drug, because trying to go without it led to a rotten night's sleep. Then they were really hooked.

All of this criticism may seem harsh to you, so we repeat that we are not antidrug simply because we are psychologists. These adverse findings have usually come from research by medical experts, not psychologists. Dr. German Nino-Murcia, the psychiatrist in charge of the sleep disorders clinic at Stanford University, said only half-jokingly: "The best treatment for insomnia is to grab patients by the feet and shake until all the medications fall out of their pockets." We are critical of sleeping drugs because a lot of research and clinical experience shows that they don't really help with sleeping problems. Some medical practitioners have accepted this and instead of prescribing sleeping drugs as such, they will prescribe an antianxiety drug "to help you sleep." We applaud their intentions but, for the reasons we explain in chapter three, they are helping their patients out of the frying pan and into the fire.

Alcohol is also a popular form of self-help for insomnia, just as it is for anxiety. Unfortunately it has the same undesirable effects as prescription sleeping drugs. You may spend time asleep, but it won't be normal, refreshing sleep. Two or three nights of excessive drinking are enough to give you rebound sleeplessness the next night. If you then reach for the bottle to get to sleep, you are developing a drinking problem. If you have been using any drugs, including alcohol, to help you sleep, we strongly encourage you to work through the suggestions in chapter three.

Bad sleep habits or environments.   As we have suggested, you should try to deliver yourself to bed in a relaxed state. Any habits that deliver you to bed in an aroused state, or not needing sleep, can contribute to insomnia.

Food and drink. Drinking too much caffeine (in coffee, tea or cola drinks) will stimulate your arousal level. Drinking too much alcohol will rob you of the important lower levels of sleep. If your tummy is rumbling from either a lack of food, too much food, or food that was too spicy or rich, sleep will be restless. However, some sensible and moderate eating might help. It has been a popular belief that carbohydrate-rich foods, such as pasta or sweets, have an arousing and energizing effect. Researchers have found the opposite is true. A meal heavy in carbohydrates, especially when they are not balanced by other food groups such as proteins, usually has a calming and even fatiguing effect. Men tend to feel relaxed and women tend to feel sleepy. Similar effects occur in children. These effects of eating lots of carbohydrates in most people were not due to hypoglycemia, which is actually a rare condition. Providing it fits within a healthy approach to eating, increasing your carbohydrate consumption in the evening may help you sleep.

What you do before bed. Other bad sleep habits may be at the root of your problem:

- Reading exciting books or watching exciting television just before bed, or even in bed, won't help.
- Postponing important discussions with your spouse until lights out won't help, especially if they turn into arguments.
- A good sexual interaction leaves most people feeling pleasant and relaxed, but if yours leave you aroused, plan them for some other time.

- Being fit helps you sleep, but a vigorous exercise workout just before sleep probably won't.
- If you worry about being safe, taking reasonable security precautions may help you relax.

Your sleeping schedule. Watch carefully how you time your sleep. Your body has its own natural rhythms of wakefulness and sleepiness, usually associated with daylight and dark. If you have irregular times for going to sleep and waking, you can throw those rhythms out of kilter. This is most obvious when you travel across time zones or change shifts at work, but some people do it to themselves by going to bed early one night and late the next. Two of the worst sleep habits are to sleep in and to nap during the day, in an attempt to catch up on sleep missed the night before. You may catch up, but at the expense of your sleep needs the next night.

Your sleeping environment.   A noisy or uncomfortable sleep environment can contribute to insomnia. Try to arrange the level of lighting and sound so that they are comfortable for you. You may be surprised how much it helps to put in earplugs if the noise in your environment is out of your control. If the noise is your spouse snoring, you may be doing him a favor if you encourage him to seek help for it. Snoring is sometimes associated with breathing irregularities during sleep that are serious health risks for the snorer.

Conditioning.   As we discuss earlier, having insomnia itself can train you to be an insomniac, long after the original cause of your disturbed sleep has gone. The more you associate being in bed with struggling to sleep, the harder it becomes for you to relax there. Eventually anything that signals that bedtime is approaching, such as brushing your teeth, can become an arousing stimulus because it warns you that the battle for sleep is about to begin again. The more you learn to worry about not being able to sleep, the more that worry will arouse you and stop

> The more you associate being in bed with struggling to sleep, the harder it becomes for you to relax there.

you from sleeping. Dr. Hauri found that 15 to 20 percent of the patients at the Dartmouth sleep clinic were naturally light sleepers who, during a period of stress, had learned bad sleep habits and become conditioned to have insomnia even after the stress was gone. If this applies to you, you will now need to reverse that conditioning by following a sleep-management program.

MANAGING YOUR SLEEP BETTER

Learn to relax physically.   Use your deep relaxation skills to help you fall asleep. A number of people have told us they get to sleep quite well following physical relaxation instructions on a cassette. If you share your bed with someone, you can listen to the tape through headphones or earplugs.

Try to have a regular bedtime, with reasonable flexibility. However, don't go to bed if you don't feel at all drowsy. Do something quiet and relaxing until you do.

If you're not falling asleep easily, don't worry about it.   Try a coping statement instead, such as the following:

> Worrying about not going to sleep is a good way of keeping myself awake. It's disappointing that I'm not asleep yet, but I can cope with that. I won't deny my disappointment, but I won't arouse myself by worrying about not sleeping. Right now I'll use my relaxation skills to relax my body and I'll focus my mind on a relaxing fantasy.

And do both of those things.

If you are not asleep after half an hour and you are becoming tense or frustrated, get up and go to another room. (If you are lying in bed relaxed and comfortable, stay there.) The same advice applies if you wake during the night and don't easily go back to sleep. Do something quiet and relaxing until you feel drowsy and then go back to bed. Repeat this procedure as often as you need to. If that means you spent an hour sitting in the lounge room reading or listening to music, that's better than spending the same hour tossing and turning in bed. Some people find a small snack helps them to go back to sleep and the research above would favor a carbohydrate snack, such as bread. Milk has been recommended in the past because it contains tryptophan, a natural sleep-inducing substance. However, some researchers now think that there isn't enough tryptophan in milk to help you sleep. Try it if you want to and decide for yourself.

Reduce alcohol, tobacco, chocolate, coffee, tea and caffeinated soft drinks in your diet, especially in the late afternoon and evening. If you think you are sensitive to caffeine, you may need to skip it altogether.

Keep fit with regular exercise. As explained above, this will help you to manage daytime stress better and reduce the fatigue that can actually make sleeping difficult or disturbed.

Don't eat heavy meals just before bedtime. You may like to gain the calming and sedating effect of a carbohydrate-rich meal, such as pasta for a main course or cake for dessert, but don't overdo the calories and do give yourself time to start digesting before bed. And we repeat our suggestion of moderate alcohol intake.

Reserve your bed for sleep (and sex if that leaves you feeling relaxed). Don't use bed as a place to worry, have important discussions or arguments, or read or watch arousing stuff. Plan those activities for other times and places.

Start a worries book: a small notebook by your bed, in which you can write down ideas or problems as they occur to you, especially in the evening or during the night. Then you can use a coping statement, such as the following:

> I expect to feel aroused if I worry about that now, but I don't have to. I have written it on my list of things to deal with tomorrow and that's as much as it is sensible for me to do now. So now I'll use my relaxation skills and a relaxing fantasy to help myself sleep.

And do it.

It may help if you jot down a brief plan of what you intend to do tomorrow, but don't be lured into doing your daytime problem-solving during your sleeping time.

Experiment with your bedroom to find the sleeping environment best for you. Vary the light level. Try different temperatures. Does some quiet music help? Most clock-radios have a sleep button that switches the radio off after an hour or so. It's a big expense, but should you change beds? We think a good waterbed is the greatest invention since sliced bread, but what do you find comfortable?

Get up at the same time each day. This is even more important than going to bed at the same time. Do not sleep in, even if you don't feel great for the rest of the day. You will only waste your sleep needs and upset your biological rhythms.

Do not nap during the day, for the same reasons. If you had a bad night's sleep, try to keep physically active rather than napping and you will help yourself sleep better the next night.

Manage your daytime stress and anxiety. Work on the rest of your anxiety-management plan. If necessary, start some systematic stress management.

Get medical advice if you think any of the medical problems listed above may be disturbing your sleep. If you have been using drugs to help you sleep, discuss our advice with your doctor and consider weaning yourself off the drugs.

Practical Exercise

From the suggestions above, pick the ones that seem likely to help you sleep better and list them below. If you are not sure whether a tip will help you, you are better off including it in your list rather than leaving it out. Try out each suggestion for at least a week before you decide it isn't helping you. It takes time to change habits.

_____

_____

_____

(continues)

_____

_____

_____

_____

RECORDING YOUR OWN RELAXATION TAPE

You will need a cassette recorder (most small ones have a built-in microphone and automatic level controls) and a sixty-minute cassette (to give you thirty minutes of uninterrupted tape time). You need somewhere reasonably quiet to make your recording so that your tape does not have distracting background noises on it. Read over the instructions below a couple of times to get a feel for them, then try recording them at a pace you think will be relaxing for you. Slow works best. Don't worry if you make a mistake or if your first try doesn't sound right. You can always rerecord all or part of your tape until you are satisfied with it.

You can change our suggested instructions to something more like what you would say, but don't change them too much. They are based on a well-proven relaxation technique. You will notice we refer to your "dominant hand" because we don't know whether you are right- or left-handed. You do, so on your tape you might feel more comfortable saying "right hand" (if you're right-handed) or "left hand" (if you're left-handed). You can make a similar substitution when we talk about "your nondominant hand."

Record the following relaxation instructions. Do not read the instructions in the parentheses out loud. Do them instead.

> To begin, I will concentrate my attention on my breathing . . . focus my attention on my breathing . . . I am going to use my breathing to help me relax, so I will concentrate all of my attention on my breathing, deliberately making it slow and deep . . . notice that breathing out is a

relaxing thing to do, letting the tension go from the muscles in my chest . . . each time I breathe out, I will feel myself relax a bit more . . . relax . . . relax . . . (Keep this up for a couple of minutes, saying "relax" at about the pace of your slowed breathing.)

Now, I'll stop thinking "relax" and concentrate on my dominant hand. The next time I breathe in, I'll think "tense" and make a tight fist with that hand . . . tense and hold the tension for a couple of steady breaths . . . the next time I breathe out, I'll think "relax" and relax my hand . . . relax . . . (keep thinking "relax" in time with your breathing) . . . even if my hand feels completely relaxed, I imagine some tension flows out of it when I tell myself to relax.

(Now repeat the instructions for this tense-and-release cycle twice more.)

Now, stop thinking "relax" and concentrate on the dominant hand. The next time I breathe in, I'll think "tense" and add the smallest amount of tension to that hand, just enough so I can feel it building up tension . . . tense . . . each time I breathe in, think "tense" and add a small amount of tension to my hand . . . (say "tense" about five times, in time with your breathing) . . . now hold that tension and keep breathing steadily . . . the next time I breathe out, I'll think "relax" and let go the smallest amount of tension from my hand, just enough so I can feel it is relaxing . . . relax . . . (say "relax" about five times, in time with your breathing) . . . even if my hand feels completely relaxed, I'll imagine some more tension flows out of it when I tell myself to relax.

(Now repeat the instructions for this gradual tense-and-release cycle twice more.)

Now I can recognize degrees of relaxation and tension better, focus my attention on the wrist on my dominant hand . . . each time I breathe out and think "relax," I can feel some tension flow out of my wrist . . . (repeat "relax" about five times, in time with your relaxed breathing) . . . now I'll concentrate on the muscles in my forearm . . . (repeat "relax" about five times) . . . now I'll concentrate on the muscles in my upper arm . . . (repeat "relax" about five times) . . . now I'll concentrate on the muscles in my shoulder . . . (repeat "relax" about five times)

Now I'll concentrate on my nondominant hand, arm and shoulder . . . each time I breathe out, I'll think, "Relax, I can feel tension flow out of those muscles" . . . (repeat "relax" about five times, in time with your relaxed breathing) . . . now I'll concentrate on my feet . . . (And so on, focusing on one major muscle group at a time. Give yourself an instruction to "relax" about five times, in time with your relaxed breathing.) . . . now my legs . . . now my back . . . now my chest . . . now my tummy . . . now my head and neck . . . now my whole body is relaxing, from head to toe . . . more and more . . . each time I breathe out, and think "relax."

(Some people like to finish their relaxation practice by imagining a relaxing and pleasant situation, instead of saying "relax." If you want to do this, you can describe your relaxing situation on your tape. Some people like to add some relaxing music. At the end of your relaxation training instructions, give yourself some instructions to bring yourself back gradually.)

Now I will gradually bring myself back . . . add a little tension to my muscles . . . breathe a little faster . . . when I'm ready, I'll open my eyes and sit up slowly, feeling refreshed and relaxed.

When you listen to your tape, set the scene to help you relax. Find somewhere quiet and comfortable, where you won't be disturbed. Have soft lighting and maybe some relaxing background music. A warm bath or shower beforehand can get you started.

—13—

How to Strengthen Social and Sexual Skills

- Social or sexual situations may be an important source of your anxiety, directly or indirectly. If so, strengthening your social and sexual skills and confidence will be an important part of your anxiety-management plan.
- Reasonably good self-esteem helps you build successful relationships.
- Strengthening social skills involves finding avenues for meeting others, introducing yourself and having social conversations.
- Making relationships more emotionally intimate involves gradually increasing the intimacy of your conversation and activities and preparing for sexual relationships.
- You will do all of this more easily, and cope with loneliness better, if you think realistically about it.
- Relationship and sexual problems require more specific suggestions to solve.

Your social and sexual relationships can be involved in your anxiety problem in several ways. They may be directly involved, if it is social or sexual situations that make you feel anxious. They may be indirectly involved, if social or sexual problems are increasing your stress levels and therefore your risk of being anxious. They may also be involved by their absence. If you lack social or sexual relationships, there is a strong likelihood you suffer from loneliness, which is in turn a common source of stress. For all of these reasons, strengthening your social or sexual skills and confidence may be an important part of your anxiety-management program.

Do I Need This Chapter?

If you're not sure whether to work on this chapter, try this checklist. Answer "yes" or "no" to the following questions.

Do you have several friends with whom you share some good times reasonably often?

Do you have one or two close friends with whom you can share confidences when you want to?

Do you attend social, sporting or fun activities reasonably often?

Are you reasonably comfortable introducing yourself to people and having social conversations?

The more times you answered "no," the more risk there is that you lack satisfactory social relationships and may be suffering some loneliness. This in turn may be increasing your stress and your risk of anxiety. But there are two important points about these questions you should consider:

1.   You may have said something like, "I don't have many friends or social activities but that doesn't matter because I am happily married." We would suggest some caution about this possibility. It would be putting a lot of pressure on your marriage to expect it to meet all of your companionship and emotional support needs. That kind of pressure can drain a marriage. It also makes you more vulnerable to any problems in your marriage, which will have more impact on you if you have no other successful relationships.

2.   Your lack of social relationships may not reflect a lack of social skills. In our discussion of social anxiety and shyness in chapter 7, we point out that socially anxious people often lack social skills, but this does not mean always. Some will say that they know quite well what to do in social situations—they can even roleplay social skills quite well in therapy with us—but they will say they are too anxious to try it in real situations. These people are usually talking themselves into their social anxiety. They will benefit more from the coping skills in chapters 10, 11 and 12 than from those in this chapter. Not sure? Then read this chapter now. If you can honestly say, "I know how to do all that" by the end, then go back and concentrate on chapters 10, 11 and 12.

SELF-ESTEEM

People who genuinely know what to do socially or sexually but tell themselves they can't do it successfully are revealing their lack of self-esteem. To have successful relationships with others, you need a successful relationship with yourself. Although we have seen a few people whose battered self-esteem has been greatly helped by their finding a successful relationship, this relationship needs a patient and caring partner who won't be put off by your lack of self-esteem.

If you don't like yourself, you won't expect others to, so you will be poor company or avoid company altogether. If you don't love yourself, in the sense of seeing yourself as lovable, you won't believe it when someone says to you, "I love you." It will go through the filter of your low self-esteem and come out as, "I want something." If you don't see yourself as sexy, in the sense of being reasonably good at giving and receiving sexual pleasure, then you won't act sexy and your negative belief becomes a self-fulfilling prophecy.

> If you don't love yourself, in the sense of seeing yourself as lovable, you won't believe it when someone says to you, "I love you." It will go through the filter of your low self-esteem and come out as, "I want something."

Not surprisingly, self-esteem (or rather a lack of it) is involved in most psychological problems, not only anxiety. Lacking self-esteem sets you up to behave in self-defeating ways and to develop problems. Having psychological problems knocks your self-esteem. So building a realistic and robust self-esteem is a part of solving many problems, including anxiety problems. A key to this is straight thinking about yourself, so chapter 11 is appropriate for you to work through.

TROUBLED MARRIAGES

In this chapter we focus on a lack of successful social or sexual relationships. You may be in a long-term relationship, such as a marriage, that has major problems. You don't lack relationships, you have a troubled one. Again, that's too big a topic for us to include in this book. There is a limit to how much you can fit into any one book and this one is going to be big enough just trying to cover anxiety-related issues. We suggest good self-help marriage books or a qualified marriage counselor. When you shop for a self-help book, be choosy. Does the author have relevant qualifications? Is the advice in the book based on scientific research, not just the author's personal experience?

FINDING FRIENDS

Finding potential friends may seem easier for young adults than it is for older adults because the majority of recognized mixing places are aimed at younger groups. However, this difference may be illusory. Other people's expectations of a relationship with you can reflect the location. Bars, dance clubs, and so on are often frequented by people looking for brief and casual relationships. If you are looking for a one-night stand, they are the places to be. You might find a casual relationship that eventually develops into a long-term one, but you should expect some disappointments along the way.

The path we recommend is slower, but much more likely to turn up longer lasting relationships. First you need to find and begin some recreational activities. They should be activities you enjoy for their own sake (you will immediately meet the recreational needs of a successfully balanced life), but through which you can expect to meet new people. A hobby that involves working alone at home refinishing furniture may be good recreation, but is unlikely to help you meet new friends, unless you combine it with going to meetings of a refinishers' club.

Stuck for ideas? Newspapers often contain suggestions, especially the ones that have a weekly guide to activities in your city. They usually list all sorts of activities and groups, indoors and outdoors, one-time and regular. Read through, using a felt-tip pen to circle anything that sounds interesting. It helps to approach this exercise in a brainstorming frame of mind. Don't leave anything out for practical or cost reasons—circle everything that looks interesting to you. Even if you later have to discard an idea, for whatever reason, it may have prompted another good idea that you would otherwise not have had. An excellent path for meeting people is adult education courses. These are offered by community centers and colleges as well as universities (where they are often part of an extension or extended university program). They can range from one-time seminars to summer schools or full-year courses, covering a range of interesting topics.

Singles' organizations have a mixed record of success as meeting places. Every time we say this we get shouted at by one or two singles' organizations, and we accept that some of them work reasonably well some of the time at helping some of their members make new friendships. But we have often been told by people who have tried singles' clubs that they can be marred by an air of desperation, that attending one felt like being on inspection in a meat market.

We suggest you treat them as you would any new activity. Try one or two, if you want to. If you do enjoy their activities and make some new friends, great! If not, discard them and try something else from your list of possible social activities. The same caution applies to commercial introduction services, some of which are obviously rip-offs. If you are required to pay a lot of money or sign any binding contracts up front, before you have had a chance to try their services, we suggest you skip them.

INTRODUCE YOURSELF

The big advantage to meeting people through sharing enjoyable activities is that you already have at least one common interest. This provides some of your conversation and good times together, beginning the process of building closeness. The disadvantage is that most people are going to the activity to do it, not primarily to meet people. Even if they are there with both recreational and social intentions, like you, they may also be a bit shy (like you). Either way, you will have to take more responsibility for initiating social contact than you might need to in a purely social setting. This is where you will need to use some basic social skills.

NONVERBAL COMMUNICATION

In all of these skills, there is an important component of nonverbal behavior. Most of your emotional impact on another person is conveyed by your nonverbal behavior, rather than by what you say. This is certainly true of social situations.

- If you look anxious or shy, you are quite likely to trigger similar feelings in the person you are talking to. On the other hand, if you look reasonably relaxed and comfortable, that helps to put the other person at ease and facilitates your conversation.

- Try to keep eye contact about half of the time. Either too little or too much can be offputting. If you find eye contact difficult, look at a spot in the middle of the other person's forehead instead.
- Try to smile at appropriate times, such as when you first meet or if something funny is being discussed. Smiling makes you look friendly.
- Speak audibly, loudly and clearly enough to be understood, without coming on too strong.
- Use a few relaxed hand gestures to animate your conversation, without imitating a windmill.

VERBAL COMMUNICATION

To start a conversation, just introduce yourself: "Hello, my name's Jane. What's yours?" You don't need anything more elaborate than that. Try to ask mostly open-ended questions. These are questions that leave most of the answer open to the other person, such as "What do you do in your spare time?" Closed-ended questions give the other person little choice as to how he will answer, such as "Do you go fishing?" He can really only answer "Yes" or "No," so he isn't contributing much to the conversation. Open-ended questions give the other person an invitation to say as much as she wants, which takes the conversational load off you. Closed-ended questions make assumptions about the other person and may reflect your interests more than his. Open-ended questions show an interest in finding out what this person is really like, rather than you imposing your assumptions or interests on her. Figure out a few and have them up your mental sleeve, ready to use:

- "What sort of work do you do?"
- "How do you fill in your day?"
- "What do you do in your spare time?"
- "What do you think about (some current topic)?"

GIVING AND RECEIVING COMPLIMENTS

When it seems appropriate, give compliments, meaning a clear statement of what you liked, such as "That's a great outfit you're wearing. It really suits you." Or, "That was a good restaurant you chose. I enjoyed that dinner, especially your company." People like to be liked and are then more likely to like you back. Don't go overboard and lay it on too thickly, or your compliments will seem unimportant. But do deliberately remark on the points in your friend or relationship that you especially like. On the other hand, accept compliments clearly and nondefensively: "Thanks, I'm glad you liked it."

Open-ended questions give the other person an invitation to say as much as she wants, which takes the conversational load off you. Closed-ended questions make assumptions about the other person and may reflect your interests more than his.

Or, "Yes, that was fun. Let's do it again soon." Do not throw compliments back into your friend's face by being defensive, by saying for example, "Oh, it's just a bunch of rags I picked up at a sale." Or, "Yes, I suppose it was OK, but I only got the name of the place from the *Good Food Guide* [ignoring your friend's compliment regarding your enjoyable company]." Ignoring or belittling compliments punishes the other person for trying to be friendly toward you. Accepting compliments does not mean you have a swelled head, only that you are capable of being friendly.

HANDLING SILENCES

During your social conversations, accept silences as a normal event. Comfortable conversation has a relaxed pace, which may include periods of silence. People often go silent because they are thinking about something. If you want to hear what he thinks, let him think. If you have both genuinely run out of conversation, relax, take your

time, and pick another open-ended
question or topic from your mental list
of possibilities.

WATCH YOUR
SELF-TALK

Ignoring
or belittling
compliments punishes
the other person for
trying to be friendly
toward you.

Beware of mind-reading, of assuming that
the other person is judging you badly or does
not like you, when you almost certainly do not have any evidence to
confirm that assumption. Unless she actually turns around and says
to your face, "You are the most boring and ugly twit I've ever met,"
you don't really know what she's thinking. The pained look on his
face may come from a toothache or the silence may result from her
shyness. Use the coping statement from chapter 10 (pages 145–155)
to manage your anxiety about meeting people and do some straight
thinking, from chapter 11, to keep your self-talk realistic and
helpful.

THREE COMMON
SOCIAL THINKING MISTAKES

There are three common mistakes that could hold you back in
making friendships. The first is to think something like "I can't get
into relationships because my last one ended." This is a common
thinking mistake of overgeneralizing.

The second is to think something like "No one could really like
me, because I am so ugly, dull, boring (or whatever)." This is
another common thinking mistake of taking things personally.
However, be willing to look at yourself realistically. Should you
improve your appearance? Do you try too hard to impress? Are you
too passive, too self-devaluing, or too aloof? Realistic self-esteem can
pinpoint goals for improvement, as well as acknowledge your
existing good points.

The third mistake is to think something like "If I try to make
friends (again), I will only be rejected and that will hurt too much

(again), so it's safer not to try." This is an example of the common thinking mistakes of overgeneralizing and imagining the worst. You can think straighter than that.

You can adapt the coping statement from chapter 10 to help you with social anxiety:

> I expect to feel anxious mixing with people and trying to make friends. I would feel bad if I made a social mistake or was rejected by someone. But I can cope with those feelings, and the chance of them happening is not a good enough reason for me to miss out on friendships or wind up lonely. So, I will choose whom to talk to, figure out what I will say to start—now, do it!

And give yourself a shove in the back and go for it.

THE MYTHS OF FRIENDSHIP

While you are making friends, beware of the influence of popular myths about friendships. These are unrealistic but common attitudes that could interfere with your success in relationships. As with other popular myths, don't ask yourself whether you believe these, but whether you are influenced by them.

Popular Irrational Beliefs about Friendship

1. Lovers are better than friends.
Well, that depends on what you had in mind. Lovers are probably better and more appropriate for sharing your sexuality with, but good friends can be at least equally good for sharing emotional intimacy.

2. Friendship should happen naturally.
We are coming to loathe the word "natural," which should mean "free of unusual influence" but is usually used to mean "habitual" or "unthinking," neither of which guarantees successful relationships. You may eventually be

habitually good at making successful relationships, but that will take a lot of deliberate practice, and even then it will require continuing effort.

3. Single people should have single friends.

Or so some couples seem to believe, since they never invite along their single friends. Security for a relationship depends mostly on its success, not on hiding it from "threats." People should have friends—current relationship status is irrelevant.

4. Close friends must be of the same sex.

Or people will suspect there's something going on. Given Kinsey's discovery of how many people have homosexual feelings and at least transient homosexual relations, this myth is really silly. Successful and valuable friendships may involve intimacy and strong commitment, without any sexual involvement. Even when some sexual feelings occur, you can choose to accept them without having to express them. This myth just cheats you of half the population as potential friends.

5. Best friends are the only worthwhile kind.

Again, it depends on what you had in mind. Best friends are important for intimacy and support. Casual friends can be at least equally good for sharing recreation and having fun. Some of them may eventually become better friends. You have to start somewhere!

6. Friends are always there.

Or they weren't "real" friends to begin with. That's a good example of black-and-white thinking. If your friends are also trying to lead a balanced lifestyle, then there will inevitably be times when they are not available to you. This is why you should have more than one friend, rather than putting such unreasonable demands on one person.

"BUT I DON'T KNOW WHAT TO SAY!"

You now have suggestions of what to say to yourself while meeting others as well as some preliminary ways to break the ice. But, you grumble, I don't know what to say to them throughout an entire conversation! A fair comment, and the solution is much simpler than you might expect. In social conversations, people generally discuss three topics. Get on top of these and you are ready for social chat with anybody.

TRIVIA

First, talk about trivia, such as the weather, sports, current affairs, politics and so on. Some shy people make life more difficult for themselves by insisting that they don't want to be like everybody else and just talk about trivia. They want to get straight into deep and meaningful discussions. This will actually scare off many people. Don't underestimate the value of trivia as conversation starters and fillers. It's emotionally safe because it is personally trivial, even though it may be genuinely interesting (at least sometimes). It provides you with nonthreatening conversation, which may be all you want with this person, at first anyway. You do not need to be an expert on trivia (unless you are determined to win board games). Read a newspaper or watch or listen to a news broadcast once a day and you will be sufficiently familiar with what's going on to have a conversation.

COMMON INTERESTS

Second, talk about your common interests, the work, recreation, hobbies, sports or mutual friends you have in common with this person. This is where open-ended questions come into their own, as the means of discovering common interests. You will often see two people meet socially, introduce themselves, chat a little about trivia, and then discover a common interest. Then they're off, set for at least an hour's worth of conversation as they swap ideas and information about their shared interest. If you want it to, such a discussion can open the way to an invitation to do that common interest together and you have a date already.

Can't find any common interests, despite trying a few open-ended questions? It is possible that you will have little in common with some of the people you meet. You can try to be friendly toward most of the people you meet, but don't expect to be friends with all of them. If this is the first time you have met this person, and you don't feel any particular need to make a success of this friendship, excuse yourself politely and move on. Start a conversation and explore the friendship possibilities with someone else.

Meeting new friends takes persistence more than anything else. It can be difficult and does involve some luck. You will meet some people you don't like or with whom you have little in common. Give yourself a pat on the back for trying and try again. On the other hand, if this person is attractive or important to you, but you are stymied by a lack of common interests, you can try to make some. Invite her to try some of your regular interests, or be willing to try some of hers, or use the search outlined above to discover some new ones that you are both willing to try.

YOU

Third, talk about yourself. We are not suggesting that you boast, which generally turns people off, but that you deliberately share some things about yourself. This means telling the other person something personal, something that you obviously would not tell just anyone. If he wants to develop a friendship with you, he will respond to your self-disclosure with a similar piece of self-disclosure. This is how relationships develop emotional intimacy. By sharing personal information, you are showing your friend that you trust her.

Don't spill out your life story after two minutes of trivia. That will really scare off potential friends. You can imagine yourself as an onion, consisting of an outer skin you would let anyone see, covering a layer you would share with most people, and then another layer you would share with fewer people, and so on, until you reach a core you would share with only one or two intimate friends, if anyone. Peel your onion slowly and watch your friend's reaction. If your friend does not reciprocate your self-disclosure, or draws the line at a certain level of closeness, recognize that that is as far as this relationship will develop, at least for now. Bear in mind the discussion of friendship myth number 5 above. Don't throw the baby out with the bathwater by abandoning this relationship. Even casual friendships are a good resource and may develop further later. In the meantime, persistent application of the suggestions above should help you to find a circle of friends.

Practical Exercise

If you have decided you need to strengthen your social skills, read over the suggestions above carefully, marking the ones you think apply to you. Some you can start on right away, such as finding possible activities through which you can meet people. Some you can start practicing right away, such as the conversational skills. Don't be afraid to practice social skills in front of a mirror or into a tape recorder. These are practical skills and you will improve with practice.

COPING WITH LONELINESS

You can't, and would not want to, work on social skills and finding relationships all the time. These are projects that are going to take some time to be successful. Meanwhile, there will be times when you are alone and at risk of being lonely. Psychologists researching in this area have defined loneliness as bad feelings that come from being alone. Transient loneliness is the everyday, brief feeling that all of us have from time to time and is not a problem. Situational loneliness is what may happen to someone who has previously had successful relationships that have been lost as a result of changes in his living situation, such as moving, separation or divorce or the death of his spouse. It may not be a problem if the person is able to follow the same steps as he used previously to make relationships. If not, then he will need to follow the steps in this chapter. Chronic loneliness is what happens to someone who has had no successful relationships, at least not for some years. If that's you, then you need to work carefully through this chapter.

> Being alone does not have to mean being lonely. Solitude is feeling good about being alone. It is valuable stress-management, particularly for people with jobs that require them to deal with other people a lot.

Being alone does not have to mean being lonely. Solitude is feeling good about being alone. It is valuable stress-management, particularly for people with jobs that require them to deal with other people a lot. People generally use their solitude to relax and reflect, to consolidate their grip on current issues or just to daydream. How you feel about anything, including being alone, depends a lot on how you think about it. So when you are alone, watch your self-talk. If you are feeling very lonely for very long, you are probably thinking unhelpfully and need to brush up on chapters 10 and 11.

A Coping Statement for Loneliness

"It is disappointing to be alone when I don't want to be and I may feel lonely then, but I can cope with those feelings. I won't deny my loneliness; it's understandable if I don't want to be alone right now. But I won't exaggerate it, either, by dwelling on it. Some time by myself can be valuable, for relaxation and reflection. If I am alone more than I want, then I should take some constructive steps to start some successful relationships."

Then give yourself a shove in the back and take some constructive steps, such as those in this chapter. However, sometimes you may need to conclude your coping self-statement with

"I am already doing as much as I can to find some successful relationships. I realize that will take some time to pay off and there is nothing I can do in that regard right now. OK, then right now I should find myself a distracting, pleasant activity to take my mind off being lonely."

Then find an activity, constructive or enjoyable, that will hold your attention. Better still, have one or two available, such as books to read or things to make or do, for those occasions when loneliness sneaks up on you.

MAKING RELATIONSHIPS EMOTIONALLY INTIMATE

So far we have given you suggestions for finding and developing friendships. That's important but, for most of us, not enough. We humans are social animals and we tend to do best when we have one or two close relationships, as well as some friendships. This does not necessarily mean you must have a couple relationship, like a marriage, although a successful couple relationship can be very good for you in many ways and is a reasonable goal to set. So, whether you are looking for one or two special friends or a life partner, we will now give you some suggestions for creating emotionally intimate relationships.

By emotional intimacy we mean sharing, closeness, support, and feelings of warmth about each other. You build intimacy by sharing good times and by good communication, involving mutual self-disclosure and acceptance. This will result in growing trust, the belief that you can count on your friend to do the right thing by you. The paradox about trust in relationships is that you have to act as though it is there: You have to make yourself vulnerable to the other person so that she can then demonstrate her trustworthiness by not letting you down. Then you have the evidence to support your trust.

> The paradox about trust in relationships is that you have to act as though it is there: You have to make yourself vulnerable to the other person so that she can then demonstrate her trustworthiness by not letting you down.

It is important to understand this. Developing any relationships necessarily involves taking the chance of being hurt, when you misplace your trust or when you want a relationship to develop further than the other person does. There is no way of being certain beforehand. If you hold yourself back from taking the chance of developing a relationship until you are certain your feelings will be reciprocated, you will never get far. You can reduce the risk by developing intimacy at a realistically gradual pace. You can demonstrate your growing commitment by giving the relationship reasonable priority. But even then you should expect to try a number of casual relationships, and to cope with some failures, in order to find a few special ones. Keep trying.

As well as increasing the intimacy of your self-disclosures gradually, you can similarly build the intimacy of your shared activities. You have probably begun by sharing structured activities—your common interests—in the company of other people. In some relationships, that is as intimate as you would want to get. For a more intimate relationship, you may choose to do some things as a couple, perhaps in the evening rather than the daytime, and eventually less structured, such as dinner together rather than tennis. But take your time, watching your friend's reaction to your initiatives, so as to develop the relationship at a mutually comfortable pace and to a mutually acceptable level of closeness.

We will consider interpersonal skills in detail in the next chapter, but for now we suggest you be assertive. Invite your friend on dates clearly and positively, without beating around the bush or inviting rejection. So it's "I would like it if you could come on a picnic on Sunday," rather than "I don't suppose you would want to do something with me some time?" And don't give up at the first refusal. He may really have something else going on. So try again, "Sorry you can't make it this Sunday. How about next weekend?"

Once again, watch your self-talk. At this stage of developing relationships, you might fall into two more common mistakes. The first is something like "If I get involved in a close relationship, I will lose all my freedom and independence." You should recognize the exaggeration in this fear. All relationships involve some loss of freedom and independence and the loss increases as your degree of mutual dependency increases. But no successful relationship, including marriage, requires the loss of all your freedom and independence. It is a cost-benefit analysis: In a successful relationship, you should feel that the cost of some lost independence is adequately compensated by the rewards of the relationship.

The second mistake is something like "Once this relationship becomes sexual, it will fail." This fear may be based on your lack of sexual experience or on your having had sexual problems or disappointments in the past. In the first case, you are making the common thinking mistake of imagining the worst, in the second case, you are making the common thinking mistake of overgeneralizing. In either case, the answer is simple: Prepare for sexual relationships. We'll give you some suggestions on this shortly.

Practical Exercise

When you have found a friendship that you would like to make more emotionally intimate, review the suggestions above, marking those that seem appropriate for you. Give yourself some practice, then push yourself to give them a try. Nothing ventured, nothing gained!

STRENGTHENING SEXUAL SKILLS AND CONFIDENCE

We are sorry to say that sex is another topic so big that it needs a book of its own to cover it properly. In the space available here, we will give you a crash course in successful sex.

The problem is that almost none of us got a sexual education. If you got a sex education, it was basically about how to make babies. That was one of the first big lies most of us heard about sex—that it was for making babies. When was the last time you had sex to make a baby? Maybe never, maybe not for a long time. Of course, there's nothing wrong with having sex to make a baby when you and your partner in a successful long-term relationship agree to do that. It's just that most of us choose to make babies only a few times in our lives, if at all. But most of us choose to have sex more often. Frequently we are being careful *not* to make a baby. So most of us are having sex most of the time not to make babies, but to make good feelings, for ourselves and our lovers, to share good feelings within a long-term relationship such as a marriage.

You did get a sex education, even if you didn't notice it at the time. Often from parents we learned embarrassment or guilt and little else; from peers we learned misinformation and jokes although, in the absence of any factual information, how do you tell which part of a joke may not be true? After these "theory" classes, most of us did our hands-on classes: petting as teenagers. You may

have learned basic baby-making, at home or at school, but we have
already pointed out how irrelevant that was. The end result of this
more or less universal sex education is a universal set of beliefs. The
trouble is, they're wrong, however popular they may be.
Approaching your sexual relationships unrealistically is no recipe for
success, so we will now describe these popular beliefs and explain
why each is untrue. In reading this list, don't smugly tell yourself
that you're not silly enough to believe any of them. Ask yourself,
instead, how much such ideas might influence your sexual behavior,
even if you can see they are silly when you read them.

Popular Myths about Sex

1. Intercourse is the adult, the best, the most important part of sex.

An overemphasis on intercourse reflects the continuing
confusion between reproduction (which generally does
require intercourse) and sexuality (which does not). It also
reflects the next myth. Since most men find intercourse
very arousing, they will naturally choose it, if allowed to
take the lead. Since most women do not find intercourse
very arousing, they can wind up pretty bored, unless they
at least share the lead. Accepting this myth makes men
worry about getting and keeping their erections and
women worry about not being aroused and satisfied by
intercourse. Research estimates vary, but only from 30 to
50 percent of women find intercourse sufficiently
physically arousing to have orgasm and then not
necessarily on every sexual occasion.

2. Men take the initiative.

Or at least we learned to expect them to, during our
lessons in petting as teenagers. Accepting this myth makes
men worry about what to do, how to do it, and when, and
it makes women worry when they are disappointed by
men's choices.

3. He is responsible for her satisfaction as well as his own.

This one is learned at the same time as myth number 2, and they both rest on the assumption that he knows what she will like. Well, only if she tells him. The only person who can usefully take responsibility for your sexual satisfaction is you. You need to know what you like and be assertive enough to ask for it. A good lover—there are no "expert" lovers—is one who will listen to and be guided by your requests.

4. Women are less interested in sex than men are. They are slower in sexual arousal and need more stimulation.

Or so it said in your handy marriage manual: "Foreplay is for the benefit of the woman." Unlike him, she needs to be warmed up. In fact, your level of sexual interest is determined mostly by how well sex works for you, by your sexual success rate. Sexually successful women—women who understand, enjoy and assert their own sexuality—are no less interested in sex nor any slower in arousal than are sexually successful men. The partner who plays a more passive role, relying on the other person's choice of technique, will usually be slower in arousal.

5. His penis is the best, most appropriate part of his body to use to stimulate her.

We are certainly not the only culture to make a fuss about penises, but that doesn't make this any less of a myth. Penises are great for receiving stimulation, as most men discover early in life. But they are poorly designed and positioned for giving effective stimulation, as most men gradually realize. Accepting this myth makes men worry about the size, shape and erectile capacity of their penises, instead of recognizing that other parts of their bodies are better designed for giving effective sexual stimulation.

(continues)

6. Her vagina is the best, most appropriate part of her body for receiving sexual stimulation.

It is this myth combined with the one before that set you up for myth number 1 and the sadly frequent overemphasis on intercourse. In fact, most of the vagina is fairly insensitive, as women who use tampons know. When women set out to stimulate themselves, to masturbate, they mostly choose to stimulate the clitoris, only occasionally to penetrate the vagina. They know what they like. If you are one of the minority of women who do find vaginal intercourse physically arousing, maybe orgasmic, that's fine, although we encourage people not to be dependent on only one form of effective sexual stimulation. If you are one of the majority of women who do not find vaginal intercourse physically arousing, at least not enough to have orgasm, don't be conned into labeling yourself as anything other than normal. Accepting this myth makes women worry about the size and shape and unresponsiveness of their vaginas and makes men worry about their sexual performance.

7. All good sex ends in orgasm. In really good sex, both partners will orgasm at the same time.

An overemphasis on orgasm, the "hunt for the big O," is only one of the unfortunate byproducts of the pop psychology of sex. Orgasms do feel great and are even healthy for you, but "musturbation" in sex is definitely bad for you. Telling yourself you "must" have an orgasm (or get an erection or lubricate your vagina or whatever) is the best way of stopping that from happening. Trying to coincide two involuntary responses like your respective orgasms is a good way of squashing your sexual fun.

8. Sex ends at 50 (or menopause or some other life point).

If sex has never been successful for you, you may be relieved to find an excuse to give it up. There is no necessary reason for sexually successful people to stop sex as they get older. You may slow down, but slowing down is not the same as stopping. There are some age-related changes in some women that can make sex uncomfortable, but these can usually be treated medically.

In place of these myths we suggest a more realistic view of sexual success: Successful sex leaves you and your sexual partner feeling good about yourselves and each other, does not offer any undue risk of harm to anyone and is unlikely to result in an unwanted pregnancy. A successful sexual relationship is one in which both partners have orgasms on most sexual occasions, somehow or other. It does not matter what sexual techniques they use, so long as these are comfortable and acceptable to both partners. And it does not matter which partner does not have an orgasm on any occasion, so long as they are both satisfied that they each have orgasms as often as they want.

Practical Exercise

Read over the popular sex myths and our definition of successful sex. If you are in a sexual relationship now, we suggest you read and discuss them with your partner. Is this realistic thinking about sex all you need? Or do you need some practical exercises for building your sexual confidence? Or some practical suggestions for solving a sexual problem? Will you try some self-help? Or is it time for professional help?

14

How to Strengthen Interpersonal Skills

- For most of us, other people are a major source of stress or anxiety.
- There are three styles for dealing with other people: submission, aggression and assertion.
- Submission may save you some confrontations but costs you bad feelings and your rights.
- Aggression may sometimes get what you want but costs you bad feelings and bad relationships.
- Assertion means dealing with others on a basis of mutual respect. It gives you the best chance of consistently getting what you want, in ways that are fair to others and that leave you feeling good about how you deal with them.
- Strengthening assertion takes some preparation and practice but can make a big contribution to managing stress and anxiety.

Being able to deal with other people skillfully and effectively can help you manage your anxiety problem in two ways:

1. Situations involving other people may be exactly what is causing your anxiety. In that case, strengthening your interpersonal skills will directly reduce your anxiety.
2. If you think about it, you will find that most of the stress in your life comes from other people. We have even found this to be true for people whose jobs look as if they should be stressful, such as police and emergency service workers. There are certainly parts of their work that are stressful, but they tell us that most of their stress comes from dealing with the people in their work. If this is true for you, then strengthening your interpersonal skills should reduce unnecessary stress in your life and therefore your risk of excess anxiety.

The key to successful interpersonal skills is assertion, although that could be misleading. Seeing assertion as a set of skills runs the risk of seeing it as a bag of tricks for getting your own way, which is unfortunately how it is often presented. Assertion is an interpersonal style. It is (or should become) your usual way of relating to others. Later we suggest assertive approaches to some common situations. But they are just examples of being assertive. As you become more skillful at assertion, you should be able to adopt an assertive approach to any situation.

NONASSERTIVE BEHAVIOR: SUBMISSION AND AGGRESSION

There are basically three ways of dealing with the people in your life, three interpersonal styles: submission, aggression and assertion.

Being submissive means keeping your thoughts, opinions and feelings to yourself, not speaking up when you should, and allowing others to walk over you, to treat you unfairly or unkindly and to rip you off. The usual motivation for being submissive is a fear of the judgments or reactions of other people if you did speak up. The submissive person expects to feel anxious if he speaks up and to feel bad if the other person reacts negatively, so he shuts up. Sometimes people are also submissive because they confuse it with being polite. In any case, the submissive person finally gives himself a poor deal. He temporarily avoids the possible bad feelings from being assertive, but then pays a higher cost in terms of lost self-esteem, recognizing how he has let himself down. In the process, he has also let someone take away some of his personal rights, and may have set up a continuing pattern in which his rights will be violated again.

Aggression involves sticking up for yourself, asking for what you want and refusing what you don't want, but it means doing that in ways that show no regard for the feelings or rights of other people. The aggressive person is out to get her way, no matter what it costs anyone else. You may be surprised to hear that aggression, like submission, is also often motivated by fear. Aggressive people can look confident, as they come barging through life like a tank, but in fact they are often motivated by a fear of losing control of the situation. Despite noisy appearances, they may be so lacking in self-confidence that they believe the only way to stand up for themselves is to come on like a ton of bricks. In a desperate attempt to stick up for themselves, they try to walk over everybody else.

The other common motivation for being aggressive is that it seems to work, at least some of the time. You can scare some of the people some of the time. However, sometimes being aggressive will earn you an aggressive reaction in return and you wind up locked in a useless and unpleasant conflict. Even when it seems to have got you your way, aggression costs. Many people feel embarrassed and guilty after an aggressive outburst. It also costs you in terms of damage to your relationships. No one likes or respects a bully.

Some people will display both nonassertive styles at different times, because they are both actually based on a lack of real confidence. These people will be submissive most of the time, bottling up more and more bad feelings because they have locked themselves into losing behavior patterns, until they finally reach volcano point and explode aggressively. Unfortunately this explosion is often directed at the wrong person, someone whom you feel less threatened by but who is not really responsible for your accumulated aggravation. Even if you are exploding at someone more appropriate, an aggressive expression of your feelings will have both of the negative costs just mentioned, to your self-esteem and your relationships. Although submission and aggression may have some short-term payoffs, by temporarily postponing bad feelings or sometimes getting you what you want, in the long term they cost you much more than they gain and are not really successful.

ASSERTION

Assertion means expressing your thoughts, opinions and feelings clearly, openly and non-defensively, and making requests and refusing unacceptable requests, but doing all that in ways that take reasonable account of the rights and feelings of other people. The underlying motivation is to show respect both for yourself and others. More than anything else, assertion is an expression of self-confidence: "I know what I think or am prepared to accept and I am confident in my ability to stand up for that, so I can afford to listen carefully to you."

It also involves realistic expectations about other people's likely reactions to your assertion and of your ability to cope with those reactions.

The big payoff for being assertive is to your self-esteem and your relationships. We want to emphasize that these are the main goals of being assertive. At the end of an assertive interaction with someone, you are able to say to yourself, "I'm pleased with how I handled that. I stood up for myself effectively, but I respected them, too." Most (but not all) other people will recognize that your assertion shows real respect for them and will eventually respond with respect for you, making your relationships more successful.

In the process, you will have maximized your influence over the other people, but we emphasize that this is a secondary goal. Being assertive gives you your best chance of getting your way, most of the time, but it does not guarantee it. You will meet some people who are rigid, inflexible, dishonest, unscrupulous or just plain stubborn. You won't always get a fair deal from the world. Despite popular myths to the contrary, there are no methods for actually controlling other people's behavior. You can sometimes get the illusion you are in control by threatening people, but threats only work while you're watching and when the threat is big. Even then, people don't like being threatened and may deliberately do the opposite of what you want, as soon as your back is turned.

If you try to control others, you are only setting yourself up for conflict and disappointment. What you really have over other people is influence, not control. Being assertive will give you consistently more influence over others and that's all you need.

PREPARING YOURSELF TO BE ASSERTIVE

Assertion is an interpersonal style, the way you deal with people all the time, and therefore it reflects how you think about others. So, an important part of preparing yourself to be more assertive is to develop an assertive frame of mind. Responsible assertion rests on two beliefs:

Assertive belief number 1:

Assertion, rather than submission, manipulation or aggression, leads to more satisfying and successful relationships and so enriches your life.

Assertive belief number 2:

Everyone is entitled to act assertively and express his or her honest thoughts, feelings and beliefs.

Practical Exercise

Read over the above two assertive beliefs and think about how they apply to you. The first is a straightforward observation, but it is important, because it is ultimately your reward for being assertive. Being assertive will take some persistent effort and sometimes will make you feel anxious. This belief tells you why it's worth those costs.

The second belief looks obvious and some people are surprised that it needs to be mentioned. But you will find many people who act as if some groups, such as children, adolescents, women or employees, should not be asserting themselves. If you are going to be responsibly assertive, that means you expect others to be assertive back to you. Real assertion involves mutual respect. What do you think?

In the space below, write how the assertive beliefs apply to your life. Do you agree? If so, do you apply these beliefs to your life? If you don't agree, why not? How does this affect how you behave toward others?

_____

_____

_____

_____

_____

_____

_____

_____

_____

_____

_____

The second belief raises a question that often arises about assertion: "But what happens when two people are assertive with each other? Don't you get stuck?" No, you don't. Two genuinely assertive people in a confrontation are much more likely to listen to each other and negotiate a mutually acceptable agreement. Two aggressive people are more likely to get stubbornly stuck. Two submissive people are more likely to compromise and reach a mutually unacceptable agreement. An aggressive versus submissive confrontation will likely result in a one-way, unfair outcome. Later we will give you suggestions on how to remain assertive with someone who is being aggressive or submissive.

Practical Exercise

How you feel about anything, including being assertive, depends a lot on how you think about it. You can help yourself become more assertive by thinking about it realistically. Here is an assertive version of the coping statement from chapter 10:

> I expect to feel anxious when I assert myself, because most people do. I will feel disappointed if I don't get the result I want, but my best chance is to stick to being assertive. I might feel embarrassed or even frightened if the other person reacts badly. I can cope with feeling disappointed or embarrassed or even frightened. The chance of feeling bad is not a good enough reason for me to surrender my rights. It's important to me to assert myself, reasonably and responsibly. So I will consider the rights and feelings of others before I assert myself. But, if it is genuinely important to me, I will assert myself.

To strengthen your assertive frame of mind, practice this coping statement often. We suggest you write it on a small card, to carry around and give yourself a refresher of assertive thinking several times a day, especially just before entering a situation in which you expect a confrontation. It's too long to use during a confrontation, although you might practice it during a thinking break (see Step 2 in "The Six Steps in Being Assertive" on pages 234–239).

LOOK FOR ASSERTIVE MODELS

In psychologists' terms, a *model* is someone whom you identify with whose successful behavior you can use as an example to guide your own. Humans actually do a lot of their learning by modeling and we recommend it to you as a way to strengthen your assertion. When you can, observe other people's interpersonal styles, how they deal with each other. Decide whether you are watching an example of assertive, submissive or aggressive behavior. This will help you to increase your awareness of the possible differences in your own interpersonal style. When you think you are watching a good example of assertion, see what you can learn from it. If he can do it, so can you.

Practical Exercise

Where can you observe interpersonal styles? At work? In malls? On the train? At home? Jot down the main points of the three styles in the definitions. Most people can identify submission easily but find it harder to distinguish assertion and aggression. Remember, the key difference is whether the person tried to respect the rights and feelings of others without surrendering his own.

We see manipulation as a form of aggression. Although the threats or coercion may be more subtle, it is still behavior aimed at serving the doer, regardless of the cost to others. Are there good examples of assertive people whom you see regularly? If so, use them as models.

REHEARSE BEING ASSERTIVE

The final part of preparing to be assertive is to pinpoint situations in which you would like to be more assertive. These could be situations that already occur frequently in your life and that you think you currently approach submissively or aggressively. Or they could be situations you have avoided until now because you didn't think you could handle them.

Practical Exercise

In the space below, write a short list of possible situations in which you want to be assertive and then rank them in order of expected difficulty for you. You should start with the easiest and work up to the most difficult, because people learn best by succeeding. For each situation, imagine yourself working through the six steps described below (page 234), but make sure that you imagine yourself being assertive. Imagine the bad ways in which others might react to your assertion and imagine yourself handling these reactions assertively too. Imagined practice does transfer well to the real world and you can take your time to get it right. When you have had a couple of imaginary practice runs, you can try it out in reality.

_____

_____

_____

_____

_____

_____

THE SIX STEPS IN BEING ASSERTIVE

We have described the process of being assertive in six steps, but this is more to help you understand it. We don't expect you to work through these steps rigidly in order. For example, you will find the first step is to listen and validate. In a conversation that lasts for more than a minute, you will probably need to do both these things several times. In the fifth step below are suggestions for thinking assertively during a conversation. In a difficult confrontation, you might need to use these thoughts often, to help you stick to being assertive. So, these six steps are more or less in the order you will usually do them, but some of them you may need to repeat as you go. With practice, they will become your interpersonal style rather than separate steps.

Step 1: Listen And Validate. Responsible assertion involves showing respect for the rights and feelings of others in the situation. If you don't give them the chance to say their piece or if you don't listen carefully, you can't respect their rights. If you won't acknowledge their thoughts or feelings as being valid for them, then you are assuming you have the right to tell others how to think and feel. If you won't listen to and validate others, you can't expect them to do that for you.

Listening looks easy. I have two ears, aren't I listening? In fact, there is a big difference between listening and hearing. *Hearing* is the involuntary process of a sound being received by your ear and transmitted to your brain as nerve signals. Hearing depends only on the sound being loud enough to grab your attention (and your not being deaf). Sometimes you will hear sounds you do not want to hear, such as distracting noises while you work or annoying noises when you want to sleep.

Listening, in contrast, is an active process of attending to and trying to understand what is being said. Here are some tips for being a good listener.

Listening Tips

- **Actively pay attention.** A trick for strengthening your listening is to pretend to be a tape recorder. When someone is saying something to you, set yourself the goal of being able to play it back when she is finished. You don't have to be able to repeat it word for word, just be able to play it back without making any important changes. Notice that we are only suggesting that you be able to play it back, not that you actually repeat everything others say to you. Setting this goal will get you actively paying attention.

- **Show that you are paying attention.** This encourages the other person to communicate with you. Face toward him, maybe lean a little toward him. Try to keep a comfortable distance between you, neither too close nor too far away, although you may have noticed this varies for people from different cultures. In a comfortable conversation, people have eye contact about half the time. If keeping eye contact makes you uncomfortable, look at his nose or forehead.

- **Don't interrupt, even if you have strong feelings about the topic of conversation.** Interrupting shows him that you are not even willing to give him a say. This often escalates a conflict. If you are finding it difficult not to interrupt, think: "Shut up! It's my turn to listen now. I'll have my say next. Listening does not mean I agree or give in, only that I respect his right to have a say."

- **Don't do all the talking.** If you don't let her get a word in, you won't hear what she has to say. This is harder if she is silent, which puts pressure on you to say something. People often use silent time to think. If you want to hear what she thinks, wait. If he is silent because he is being submissive, look at our suggestions later about how to stay assertive with someone being submissive.

- **Listen to the unspoken message.** Not everyone has had the chance to learn to be assertive, so they won't necessarily be open about their feelings. But they will give you nonverbal clues about their feelings, such as their facial expressions, how they talk rather than what they say, and their body language. In fact, these nonverbal clues usually tell you more about a person's feelings than any words do. Be careful. When you read these nonverbal clues you are mind-reading, guessing what the other person thinks or feels. Mind-reading is popular but easily mistaken. So share your guess and check it by saying, for example, "You don't look very happy about this, Joan. Is there something you want to say?" If your guess is wrong, she can tell you. You have done your assertive bit by inviting her to share her feelings.

Validating is how you express your respect for the other person's rights and feelings. You simply show that you accept that what he has said is true for him. In principle, validating is simple. For example: "Yes, George, I can see you are angry about this." "Okay, Nguyen, I understand you think we should close on Saturdays." People often find it difficult to validate because they confuse it with agreeing or giving in. It is neither of these things. It only amounts to saying: "I understand that is how you think or feel, because you just said so and you are the world's expert on your thoughts and feelings."

Validating is a powerful technique for defusing conflict assertively. Validate the other person first, then have your say: "Right, Mark, I understand you want us to paint it green and I can see why you think that's a good idea. However, I still think blue would be a better color for this job." Here are some tips to help you validate.

Validating Tips

- **Validate clearly, promptly and nondefensively.** You won't always understand why someone thinks or feels as she does and you don't need to. It's enough to show that you understand how she thinks or feels. For example: "Yes, I can see that's how you think about it. It's not how I think about it, but I see it's how you do."

- **Don't make excuses to defend yourself.** This is most likely when you have had an impact on someone that you did not intend. For example, you meant to help your friend but in fact you made things more difficult for him. He is now angry at you and you are tempted to justify yourself. Don't, it only makes things worse. You can still validate, while making your real intentions clear. For example: "I can see I made it harder for you and I understand that makes you angry. I meant to help, but I can see I didn't."
- **Don't tell other people how to feel.** Telling someone that it isn't "logical" to feel as she does implies she is silly for having her own feelings. Reassuring someone that everything will turn out okay implies he is silly for feeling bad now. All you are doing is making them feel bad about feeling bad. It's much more helpful just to validate.

Step 2: Think about the Situation. Responsible assertion involves flexibility, choosing to assert yourself only when your personal rights are genuinely threatened, as distinct from situations that are just not how you would like them to be. It means not being unnecessarily assertive and not being overconscious of your rights. For each situation, try to answer these three questions:

- What are the rights of all of the people in this situation? Theirs? And mine?
- Are my rights really threatened here?
- Is this a situation in which it's genuinely important to me to assert myself?

Only you can answer the last question, because your decision will reflect your personal values, interests and beliefs. An issue important to you may be unimportant to someone else and vice versa. If you decide that a situation is just unpleasant or inconvenient but not worth asserting yourself over, forget it. If you have trouble doing that, use the coping skills in chapters 10 and 11.

On the other hand, if you decide this is a situation in which you want to be assertive, go on to the next step.

Both this and the next step involve a fair amount of thinking. That's important if you want to assert yourself responsibly and effectively. But in a confrontation, you may feel under pressure to say something quickly. Don't. A hasty response is more likely to be one you will regret later, as having been submissive, aggressive or off the real issue. You have a perfect right to think things over for a reasonable time, so use it.

First, say to yourself, "I don't have to rush in. I can give myself time to think about the situation." Second, tell the others what you are doing: "Wait a minute, please, I'd like to think about this so I can give you my considered response." If someone else has trouble respecting your right to think, that's her problem.

Step 3: Figure Out How You See the Situation.   At this stage, you will plan your initial assertive response. Later we will give you some suggestions on how to assert yourself under different circumstances. Those suggestions should help you plan your assertion. Meanwhile, take time to decide what is really the important issue for you and assert yourself on that. You can be tempted to assert yourself on some other, more obvious or less personal issue. For example, your spouse has bought something big without consulting you. It might be less threatening to complain it's the wrong color, but that's not really the issue for you. If you assert yourself on the wrong issues, you may get the wrong change. Having figured out what you will say, imagine how the others are likely to respond. Figure out what you could say next, sticking to being assertive.

At this step, you set your goals for assertion in this situation realistically. We emphasize the main goal of being assertive is just that—to see yourself being responsibly assertive. A possible second goal is to influence others to change some part of their behavior. But only set that goal when you think there is a reasonable chance of obtaining it. Aiming to change the behavior of people who are obviously not going to change only sets you up for disappointment.

Step 4: Assert Yourself. When it's your turn to speak, make your initial assertive response. Try to stick to your assertive plan, but do listen to others to see if their responses suggest a change in your approach. Request more time to think if you want it. If that puts you under pressure to respond quickly, again think: "Relax; I have a perfect right to think about this." If someone else has trouble with that, that's his problem.

Step 5: Think Assertively. As the discussion proceeds, you can help yourself stick to being assertive by giving yourself brief instructions.

- If the other person becomes upset or angry, say to yourself, "Stay calm, I don't have to get upset. If she wants to, that's her problem."
- If you become upset or angry, say to yourself, "Relax; I'm in control." Back this up with a calming response (from chapter 12).
- If you or someone else start to wander off the topic or to introduce some other issue, say to yourself, "Stick to the issue; don't get sidetracked," and then you say, "I can see that (the new issue) is important to you, so let's discuss it next, but first I would like to finish this (the present issue)."

Step 6: Review the Situation Afterward. Later, when you have time to yourself, review how your assertion went. If you were successful, which means only that you were able to stick to being responsibly assertive, not whether you got anyone else to change his behavior, give yourself a pat on the back.

Similarly, being unsuccessful means you were not able to stick to being assertive. At some point you became submissive or aggressive. Try to identify that point and what you did wrong. Imagine how you could have handled it assertively instead. Then get on with life. No moping about it.

SUGGESTIONS FOR ASSERTION IN DIFFERENT SITUATIONS

Back in Step 3, you plan your initial assertive response. The form of that will vary from situation to situation. We will now give you some suggestions for being assertive in some commonly occurring situations, but these are *suggestions* for developing your assertive style, not rigid instructions.

SITUATION: SPEAKING UP

This is the most basic form of assertion—saying clearly, promptly, calmly (if firmly) how you feel or what you think. The key is to use I-language statements, such as "I feel angry about not being consulted about a decision that affects me directly" or "I would like our next vacation to be at the beach." Even though basic assertion is simple, it is the form of assertion most used for self-expression.

Let us make an important point now. If you have strong feelings of any kind, you do not have a choice about whether you share them. Most feelings are expressed involuntarily, in nonverbal cues such as the expression on your face, how you speak rather than what you say, and your body language. Whether we like it or not, we give off the vibes and other people will read them and guess how we feel. Your real choice is never "Will I share my feelings here?" It's always "How will I share my feelings here?" We suggest you share your feelings openly and assertively, by announcing them: "I feel worried about meeting these new people this evening." This open expression of your feelings is called *leveling*. It is all the more important if you are trying to discuss something or solve a problem. Unstated feelings will interfere with, and perhaps completely block, any attempt at negotiation or problem-solving. The rule of thumb is feelings first, problem-solving second. If your strong feelings have been triggered by the person you are talking to, it's even more important that you deal with them first. So we will describe that next.

SITUATION: SOMEONE'S ACTIONS ARE STRONGLY INFLUENCING YOUR FEELINGS

This is one of the most important and useful forms of assertion because it deals with the emotional side of relationships. You will usually find it is this aspect of relationships that is likely to be a source of stress or anxiety for you. Being able to tell others, assertively and constructively, how their behavior is affecting you is one of the most useful interpersonal skills.

The basic form for stating how someone else's actions affect you is

When you do X, the effect on me is Y, and I feel Z.

This formula feels awkward to everybody while they are learning it. But with some practice, you should find it becomes a good communication habit. So be willing to persist with it for a while. Here's an example: "When you did not pass on that message, I missed an important appointment and I feel angry." Now let us show you how that leveling statement was put together.

When you do X. The first part, "When you do X . . . ," is a simple description of the other person's actions, that anyone else could have seen or heard. In our example, this is "When you didn't pass on that message . . ." The other person will know exactly what he has done to affect you. Don't be vague, such as "When you don't do your job . . ." This leaves the other person guessing which part of her job you think she hasn't done. Don't make interpretations, such as "When you can't be bothered passing on my messages . . ." People will usually just deny your interpretations. Don't overgeneralize, such as "When you never pass on my messages . . ." Overgeneralizations are rarely true and they invite the other person to find exceptions—"I gave you a message last week"—rather than deal with your present complaint. Don't assassinate characters, such as "You are lazy and unreliable . . ." Telling someone you think he has a bad character usually gets you a defensive reaction. One of the advantages to leveling is that it gives people precise information. You are telling him exactly what he has done that has affected you.

The Effect on Me Is Y.   The middle part of the statement—"the effect on me is Y"—is a simple description of the direct effects of her behavior on you. In our example, this is "I missed an important appointment . . ." Here, the direct effect of the other person's behavior was to make you miss an appointment. This is often the hardest part of a leveling statement to figure out, because you are looking for a direct effect other than on your feelings. You are going to add your feelings in the third part of the leveling statement. Here you are looking for other direct effects.

The way to find the possible direct effect on you is to go to your feelings and ask "Why?" In our example, you would ask, "Why did I feel bad about that message not being passed on? Because it made me miss an important appointment, that's why." And there you would have found the Y part of your leveling statement. If you cannot find a direct effect on you of the other person's behavior, you probably should not be leveling. After all, if his behavior has not directly affected you, what right have you to comment on it?

This does not contradict our advice above about the impossibility of trying to keep strong feelings to yourself. It does guide you as to how you share those feelings. If the other person's actions have directly affected you, then level with an X-Y-Z statement. If the other person's actions have strongly affected your feelings but not directly affected you, then level by just speaking up, by making an "I-statement."

The I-Statement.   For example, on hearing that your son got drunk at a party last week, you feel upset. Since his getting drunk did not directly affect you, you don't level with an X-Y-Z. You do speak up: "I think getting drunk is not a good idea because I believe it damages your health." By leveling with an I-statement rather than lecturing with a you-statement, you have had maximum influence— and that's what assertion is about.

And I Feel Z.   The third part—"and I feel Z"—is a simple description of your feelings as a result of the other person's actions.

In our example this is "and I feel angry." Remember that you don't really have a choice about whether you share your feelings, only how. You can adjust how personal you make your leveling statement. With a casual friend or coworker, you might only level that you feel bad about something. With your spouse or a close friend you might give more details of your feelings. But you will share your feelings, whether or not you want to. So we suggest you do it openly and assertively.

Try to be accurate about both the flavor and intensity of your feelings. If you feel angry, don't say "a little annoyed." If you feel terrified, don't say "a bit scared." If you make the situation seem unimportant to you, the other person may also see it as unimportant.

There are three other points about leveling. First, have you heard of the KISS principle? KISS stands for "Keep it simple, stupid!" That's a good rule for all your assertion. You are trying to communicate, not conduct a memory test. Keep your leveling and all your assertive messages short enough for the other person to track easily. If necessary, make several statements rather than a long, complicated one.

Second, don't hit back. If someone hurts you, you'll be tempted to hurt back. You might briefly enjoy your revenge but only at a cost to the relationship. Practice leveling and you will find there is nothing anyone in your life can do that you can't level about. In a conflict, the real winner is the one who sticks to being assertive.

Third, do level about good feelings. If you only share your bad feelings, you are not a very rewarding person for others to know. Leveling about good feelings strengthens relationships.

Practical Exercise

Leveling is such an important interpersonal skill that we suggest you pause now and work on it. Identify some situations in which other people have had a big impact on your feelings and write those down below. Following the guidelines above, figure out now how you could have leveled each time: "When you did X the effect on me was Y and I feel Z." Remember, if you can't identify a direct effect on you other than on your feelings, you should not level with an X-Y-Z statement. If the situation did involve strong feelings for you, then speak up, leveling with an I-statement. Do remember to level on some good feelings, too.

Situation 1:

_____

_____

_____

_____

_____

When you do X:

_____

_____

The effect on me is Y:

_____

_____

And I feel Z:

_____

_____

Situation 2:

_____

_____

_____

_____

When you do X:

_____

_____

The effect on me is Y:

_____

_____

And I feel Z:

_____

_____

Situation 3:

_____

_____

_____

_____

(continues)

When you do X:

_____

_____

The effect on me is Y:

_____

_____

And I feel Z:

_____

_____

SITUATION: MAKING REQUESTS

It is quite common to follow a leveling statement with a request. You have told the other person what you did not like about her behavior. Now ask for the behavior you want instead. People are sometimes reluctant to make requests. "Oh, I couldn't ask her to do that; she might not want to." Notice the assumption is that, if you ask someone to do something, he must do it. Nonsense. You have a perfect right to make requests because other people have a perfect right to refuse your requests. The refuser must also be willing to bear any consequences of refusing, but she has the right to refuse. If you want someone to do something, the simplest and often most effective way of getting him to do it is to make a request.

Make your requests clear and precise, so that the other person knows exactly what you are asking. Vague requests set you up for dispute over whether they were met. Make your requests for observable behaviors, so there can be no doubt as to whether it has happened. Try to be positive and nondefensive in your manner, by simply being courteous. You do have the right to make requests and we trust yours is a reasonable one. You should also have positive content. This means to ask the other person to do something you want, not to stop doing something you don't want. Asking someone to stop doing something focuses on negative feelings and does not tell her what you want instead. Go straight to what you want instead and ask for that. While you are making your request, try to make reasonable eye contact and speak clearly and audibly. For example, you might request, "Would you please bring the car around to the front now," rather than, "I don't suppose you would like to help" (defensive and vague), or "When are you going to quit being lazy" (aggressive, character-assassination, vague).

SITUATION: REFUSING REQUESTS

As we just said, you have a perfect right to refuse requests that are unacceptable to you, as long as you are also prepared to accept any consequences that may flow from your refusal. Make your refusals clear, so that the other person is in no doubt about your intentions. Again, be nondefensive. You do have the right to refuse requests. If you want to, offer an explanation for your refusal, but you are not necessarily obliged to do so. Most importantly, refuse promptly. If you are silent after receiving a request, it is easy for the other person to misinterpret your silence as acceptance of his request. If you later announce your refusal, his reaction may be all the stronger because he thought you had accepted. If you are not sure about whether to refuse a request, say so promptly. For example, "Wait a minute, please, I would like to think about your request before I answer." If you want to take longer than a minute or two to consider your reply, give the other person an indication of when you will have an answer: "I'll let you know after I have checked my calendar (or before lunch or whenever)." Again, try to make eye contact and use clear, audible speech. For example, you might refuse the previous request: "No, I'm sorry but I can't help you with the car right now. I have something else to do," rather than, "Why should I?" (defensive) or "Well, I might get around to it later" (when you really don't intend to).

If someone makes a request that is unacceptable to you, or if you refuse an unacceptable request from someone else, you may negotiate. You can each make counter-requests or counter-offers until you arrive at a mutually acceptable agreement. There is a key to successful negotiation: Ask yourselves what you really want. For example, you might begin by saying you want the car on Saturday night. Then ask yourself, "Why? What for?" With a bit of thought you will realize what you really want is transport. Having the car is only one possible solution and there will be others. Figuring out what people really want usually makes a number of solutions possible. Among them there will usually be one that suits everybody. That's the outcome of a successful negotiation, an answer that suits everybody.

SITUATION: DISAGREEING WITH SOMEONE ELSE'S POINT OF VIEW

The key here is to recognize the other person's point of view specifically, but without surrendering your own. The basic form is "I see that's what you think; it's not how I see things." By first validating the other person's point of view you show respect for her. By sticking to your guns, you also show respect for yourself. For example: "I can see that you would like to have our next vacation at the beach, but I think going to the mountains would suit the whole family better."

SITUATION: DEALING WITH A PERSISTENT PERSON

Responsible assertion involves not squashing others unnecessarily. So, begin with the minimum amount of assertion necessary, escalating to a firmer level only if your previous attempt was not sufficient. With someone who is being unreasonably persistent, such as a pushy salesperson, you can just keep repeating your assertive message over and over again. This technique, sometimes called the "broken record," can be effective in getting rid of pests. But because of the risk of it becoming aggressive, you should use it only as a last resort. For example, he says, "Would you take care of my customers tomorrow, Carla?" You reply, "No, Jake, I don't want to." He says, "But there's a really great game on that I want to see and I know you aren't interested in football, so why not?" You reply, "No, Jake, I can see you really want to go to your football game, but I don't want to work on Saturday. I have my own plans." He says, "Don't be a rat. Whatever you've got going can wait, but this game only happens once a year." You reply, "Jake, when you won't take a polite 'No' for an answer and keep pestering me like this, you're trying to interfere in my private life and that annoys me. I'd like you to ask someone else to take care of your customers."

SITUATION: SOMEONE SAYS ONE THING, BUT DOES SOMETHING ELSE

The key here is to objectively describe the other person's words and actions, pointing out the contradiction between them. It takes the general form: "You said you would do this, but in fact you have done that." If it is appropriate, you can add a request for change: "I would like you to do this now, please." Do not fall into the trap of interpreting the other person's motives or indulging in character-assassination: "You lazy twerp, you only said you would clean up to get me to mow the lawn." Stick to an objective description of the other person's observable words and actions: "You said you would clean up while I mowed the lawn, but you haven't done a thing. I would like you to clean up now, please."

SITUATION: ASSERTING YOURSELF WITH SOMEONE BEING SUBMISSIVE

The risks here are that you may feel sorry for the submissive person and back off into being submissive yourself, or you may find his submissiveness so frustrating that you become aggressive. In any case, his submissiveness may lead to you agreeing about something he does not genuinely accept and may not adhere to later. The key here is to level about how you feel about his behavior, adding a request for change if you want to. But stick to your assertion.

The two kinds of submissiveness most difficult to handle are crying and withdrawal. Although crying is sometimes manipulative, it's usually best to take it as genuine and to validate the other person's distress. But then stick to your assertion. For example, you might say, "I can see you're upset about this and I would feel bad about it, if I were in your shoes. Still, we did agree that it was going to be done that way and I think you should stick to that agreement." If the other person seems too distressed to continue with the discussion, take time out from it. Make sure to set a specific time to return to the discussion.

Withdrawal usually takes the form of silence accompanied by lots of body talk that expresses bad feelings. Again, reflect and validate the other person's apparent feelings, while giving her room to speak if she wants to. For example, you might say, "It looks to me as if you feel angry about this, and I can see why the situation would make you feel like that. But we do have to work out a solution that suits us both. So I'd appreciate knowing what you think." For both crying and withdrawal, the advantage to your leveling is that you are giving the other person a good example of how to express her feelings more constructively.

SITUATION: ASSERTING YOURSELF WITH SOMEONE BEING AGGRESSIVE

This is the situation most feared by people who have previously been submissive but are now trying to be more assertive. "But what will I do if she gets angry?" Well, let's get one thing clear. If the person you are asserting to does get angry, you won't die. You probably will feel embarrassed, awkward or even frightened, but that's all. Use a coping statement (see chapter 10) and think straight about being assertive (see chapter 11).

Unless you are fortunate enough to be asserting yourself with someone who has also learned about assertion and therefore knows how to respond in kind, when you do assert yourself, you will often get a defensive response, whether sullen submission or hostile aggression. No matter how reasonable your assertion may be or how well you may do it, to an untrained person it will probably first appear to be an attack, and he will probably be defensive. That's not a good reason for you not to be assertive, but it is a good reason for you to expect a defensive response at first and be prepared to handle it assertively.

If the other person looks or sounds angry but isn't saying so, reflect and validate her apparent feelings. This invites her to level about them so they can be dealt with openly first. Then stick with your original assertion. For example, "You seem angry about this and I can see why you might feel like that. But, I still think you should pass on my messages, like we agreed."

If the other person responds with personal abuse or by raising other issues to attack you, don't get sidetracked into a slinging match or onto red herrings. Still reflect and validate his apparent feelings, but stick to your assertion. For example, he says, "Well, it's typical of your rigidity that you want your messages right away, like you always want your letters in duplicate." You reply, "I can understand you feel angry about this, but the issue I'd like to settle now is reliably getting my messages. If there's a problem about copying my letters, let's discuss that next."

If the other person is aggressively trying to get you to back down on some point, use the technique above of specifically recognizing her point of view while sticking to yours. If the other person's argument rests on unstated assumptions that you think are questionable, point out her underlying assumptions and your disagreement. For example, you might say, "I can see that your suggestion of painting the house ourselves would save us money, but you are assuming we can do a professional-looking job, and I don't think that's true."

Some people respond aggressively to your assertion by asking questions or trying to debate the issue with you. As a rule, don't answer questions while asserting, except in the rare case that some further information is genuinely called for. A question is more likely to be an attack on you and should be reflected as such. For example, he says, "Well, did you always stick to the plans when you were working in the front office?" You reply, "It sounds to me as if you think I am asking higher standards of work from you than I would from myself. Is that the problem?"

Don't be drawn into a debate, a verbal competition in which someone must lose. Reflect the other person's feelings and stick to your original assertion. For example, she says, "It does seem to me that there is an important principle here, about deciding the priority of different office tasks and who decides those priorities. Since I have been here longer than you, I think I should decide priorities." You reply, "I can understand you feel angry about this, but I'm not going to argue principles with you. If they are important to you, let's discuss them at the next staff meeting. Right now, I'm concerned that you have not passed on my messages as we agreed."

Practical Exercise

Now complete the exercise we began in the section on practicing being assertive (see page 229). You should have a short list of situations you want to handle more assertively. Working through the six steps in being assertive and following our guidelines for being assertive in different situations, plan your initial assertive approaches. Imagine how the others might react, usually defensively, at least at first, and figure out how you can stick to being assertive. When you have had several practice runs in your imagination, try it out in the real world. Gradually but deliberately, make assertion your interpersonal style.

═══15═══

Anxiety and Suicide

- There is a disturbingly high mortality rate associated with anxiety problems, reflecting unexpectedly high rates of heart disease and suicide, especially but not only associated with panic problems.
- It is not yet clear whether this is a direct effect of anxiety problems or the indirect result of health-damaging behavior or depression caused by anxiety problems.
- You can take practical steps to reduce your risk of heart disease.
- If you are thinking of suicide, we encourage you to consider other options for solving your problems first, because there is a high risk that suicide will be a mistake.

In chapter 2 we report the disturbing finding that anxiety is associated with a higher rate of mortality than would be expected. Patients with anxiety problems, especially but not only panic problems, suffer an unexpectedly high rate of heart disease and suicide. Suicide has long been recognized as a risk associated with depression. But these researchers compared a group of anxious

We do believe in approaching problems realistically. Since there seem to be real risks of heart disease and suicide associated with anxiety problems, we believe we should discuss these with you factually and encourage you to do something constructive about them.

patients with a matched group of depressed patients and found that the suicide rates for anxious patients were equal to or slightly higher than for the depressed patients.

We are not discussing these findings to make you feel worse about having an anxiety problem. We do believe in approaching problems realistically. Since there seem to be real risks of heart disease and suicide associated with anxiety problems, we believe we should discuss these with you factually and encourage you to do something constructive about them.

These are new research findings and we really don't understand them yet. It is possible that anxiety itself is a direct threat to your health, perhaps by causing undesirable biological changes in your body. There is already research that shows that excessive anger does this. Or it is possible that anxiety affects your health indirectly in at least two ways. First, we have previously reported that anxiety is associated with drug-dependence problems, including abuse of alcohol and other drugs. So maybe it is the overuse of these drugs that damages your health. From our work in health psychology, we know that anxiety is often a trigger for health-damaging behavior, including smoking and unwise eating and drinking, which in turn contribute to unhealthy weight. Maybe anxiety damages your health by triggering these unhealthy behaviors.

Second, we also describe the association between anxiety and depression in chapter 1. Although these two states do differ in some important ways, they also overlap a lot. It is possible that, at least for some people, long-term problems with anxiety lead to depression and it is this depression in turn that makes these people a suicide risk. We are confident that future research will answer some of these questions and make clearer just how anxiety threatens your health.

But you do not need to wait for that research before you take some sensible steps.

PROTECT YOUR HEALTH

By now, you are presumably working on your personal plan for managing your anxiety problem. Keep it up. Steady progress should reduce any direct health risks from anxiety. It will also help you to adopt a healthier lifestyle, especially if anxiety has been triggering health-reducing behavior for you.

THE WARNING SIGNS OF SUICIDE

We know that many depressed people will have thoughts about suicide and some of them will attempt it, sometimes successfully. They are more likely to try it when they feel especially hopeless about the future: "Not only is my life a mess now, but it's never going to get any better." Since we don't yet understand the link between anxiety and suicide, we don't know if it involves similar thoughts, but that seems quite possible.

So you should be watching your self-talk for similar ideas about your anxiety problem. "Not only is my anxiety problem making my life a miserable mess, it's never going to get better. Nothing I try has ever helped or ever will. I and the important people in my life would be better off if I were dead." If you are having thoughts like those, we strongly suggest you reread chapter 11. Go back to chapter 11 and actively test your self-talk about suicide. Figure out some more helpful thoughts and try those for a while.

CONSIDER THE ALTERNATIVES

We are not automatically opposed to the idea of suicide. We can imagine some circumstances under which it might be a reasonable option, such as having an incurable, painful and progressive illness. Situations like these are at the center of the current debate about euthanasia. The problem with suicide is that most of the people who seriously consider it are really not in such desperate and insoluble situations. At the time, they believe they are and that's why suicide seems a plausible solution to them. It seems to offer the only end to their suffering. But that assessment both of their situation and of their future is a clear example of unrealistically negative thinking.

Talking with people who made genuine attempts at suicide but survived, you will find that later they nearly all decide that their attempt was a mistake. They understand why it seemed to make sense at the time, because of how they were feeling and thinking, but later they realize how mistaken their thinking was. So the mistake rate in choosing suicide seems to be very high. The problem is, if your suicide is successful, it's a mistake you can't undo.

So we suggest that if you consider suicide as a possible option, also consider its own pros and cons: immediate cessation of suffering on the one hand, but hurt to those left behind, total loss of future enjoyment, and so on, on the other hand. Then we suggest you consider your other options because, dollars to doughnuts, there will be some. By now you will realize we are rather skeptical about some of the popular treatments for anxiety problems, especially the antianxiety drugs. If you have had these prescribed for you and found that they did not really help, maybe even caused you other problems, that was bad luck. The doctor who prescribed them for you almost certainly believed they would help, because he gets a lot of propaganda from drug companies. But that's not your fault. Now that you have the chance to try a research-based, drug-free plan for managing anxiety problems, take your time to give it your best shot.

> The problem with suicide is that most of the people who seriously consider it are really not in such desperate and insoluble situations.

A similar caution applies to self-help. It isn't for everybody. By now you will know how much there is in an anxiety-management program. Your difficulty in following self-help may be what is prompting you to think of suicide. Since there is a high chance that choosing the option of suicide will actually be a mistake for you, as it is for most people, it makes sense for you to try some of your other options first. If you are seriously considering suicide, perhaps because self-help has been unsuccessful or too difficult for you, we strongly encourage you to talk it over with someone. We recommend a qualified clinical psychologist, one who (in the United States) is board certified by the American Board of Clinical Health Psychology. In Canada, look for a psychologist who is accredited by the Canadian Psychological Association or who has a postgraduate qualification in clinical psychology.

Since there is a high chance that choosing the option of suicide will actually be a mistake for you, as it is for most people, it makes sense for you to try some of your other options first.

But if you can't talk to a clinical psychologist, try some other counselor or mental health professional. In an emergency, call one of the telephone counseling services. You owe it to yourself and the important people in your life to discuss and try all of the options for solving your problems before the final one.

Practical Exercise

Does anxiety trigger health-reducing behavior in you? Once you are managing your anxiety better, what steps will you take to improve your healthy lifestyle? When do they start? Have you been thinking of suicide? Have you been having hopeless thoughts about your future? Is it time you actively considered your other options for solving your problems? Is it time you discussed this with someone else? Is it time you got some professional help? Who and when?

If you are considering suicide, look back at chapter 11 and try to determine what your unhelpful thoughts are. Then work through a Questioning Your Thoughts exercise to find more helpful thoughts and constructive plans.

Resources

Agoraphobics In Motion (A.I.M.)
1719 Crooks
Royal Oak, MI 48067–1306
248-547-0400

Al Anon Family Group
Headquarters, Inc.
1600 Corporate Landing Pkwy.
Virginia Beach, VA 23454–5617
888-4AL-ANON
www.al-anon.alateen.org/

Alcoholics Anonymous
800-640-7545
www.alcoholics-anonymous.org/

American Academy of Child and Adolescent Psychiatry
3615 Wisconsin Ave., N.W.
Washington, D.C. 20016
202-966-7300
www.aacap.org

American Counseling Association
801 N. Fairfax St., Suite 304
Alexandria, VA 22314
800-326-2642
www.counseling.org

American Psychiatric Association
Public Affairs Office
1400 K St., N.W., Suite 501
Washington, D.C. 20005
202-682-6220
www.psych.org

American Psychological Association
750 First St., N.E.
Washington, D.C. 20002
202-336-5800
helping.apa.org

American Self-Help Clearinghouse
Northwest Covenant Medical Center
25 Pocono Rd.
Denville, NJ 07834
800-367-6724 (in NJ)
201-625-9565 (outside NJ)
www.cmhc.com/selfhelp/

Anxiety Disorders Association of America
11900 Parklawn Drive, Suite 100
Rockville, MD 20852
301-255-2200
Fax: 301-231-7392
www.adaa.org

Association for Advancement of Behavior Therapy
305 Seventh Ave., 16th Floor
New York, NY 10001
212-647-1890

Bureau of Alcohol and Drug Programs
976 Lenzen Ave., 3rd Floor
San Jose, CA 95126
408-299-6141
Fax: 408-279-1843

Council on Anxiety Disorders
Route 1, Box 1364
Clarkesville, GA 30523
706-947-3854;
Fax: 706-947-1265

Freedom From Fear
308 Seaview Ave.
Staten Island, NY 10305
718-351-1717
www.freedomfromfear.com

The Johns Hopkins University
The Johns Hopkins Medical Institutions
   Anxiety Disorders Clinic
600 N. Wolfe St., Meyer Room 115
Baltimore, MD 21287
410-955-5653

NAMI
Colonial Place Three
2107 Wilson Blvd., Suite 300
Arlington, VA 22201-3042
800-950-NAMI
www.nami.org

Narcotics Anonymous
World Service Office in Los Angeles
P.O. Box 9999
Van Nuys, CA 91409
800-4-HELP-NA, 818-773-9999
Fax: 818-700-0700
www.wsoinc.com/

National Anxiety Foundation
3135 Custer Dr.
Lexington, KY 40517-4001
606-272-7166

National Mental Health Association
1021 Prince St.
Alexandria, VA 22314-2971
703-684-7722 or 800-969-NMHA
www.nmha.org

National Panic/Anxiety Disorder News, Inc.
1718 Burgandy Pl
Santa Rosa, CA 95403
707-527-5738
www.npadnews.com

National Mental Health Consumers' Self-Help Clearinghouse
1211 Chesnut St., Suite 1207
Philadelphia, PA 19107
800-553-4539 or 215-751-1810
www.libertynet.org/~mha/cl_house.html

NIMH Anxiety Disorders Clinic
National Institutes of Health
Clinical Center Building 10
4th Floor Outpatient Clinic
Bethesda, MD 20892–1368
301-496-4874

Obsessive Compulsive Foundation
9 Depot St.
Milford, CT 06460
203-878-5669
pages.prodigy.com/alwillen/ocf.html

Phobics Anonymous
P.O. Box 1180
Palm Springs, CA 92263
619-322-COPE

Recovery, Inc.
802 N. Dearborn St.
Chicago, IL 60610
312-337-5661
Fax: 312-337-5756
www.recovery-inc.com

Further Reading

American Psychiatric Association. *Diagnostic & Statistical Manual of Mental Disorders DSM-IV-TR, 4th ed.* Washington, D.C.: American Psychiatric Press, 1987.

Andrews, G., R. Crino, C. Hunt, L. Lampe and A. Page. *The Treatment of Anxiety Disorders.* New York: Cambridge University Press, 1997.

Barlow, D. H. *Anxiety and its Disorders.* New York: Guilford Press, 1988.

Barlow, D. H., and J. A. Cerny. *Psychological Treatment of Panic.* New York: Guilford Press, 1988.

Barlow, D. H., ed. *Clinical Handbook of Psychological Disorders: A Step-by-Step Treatment Manual.* New York: Guilford Press, 1994.

Beck, A. T., M.D., and G. Emery, Ph.D. *Anxiety Disorders & Phobias: A Cognitive Perspective.* New York: Basic Books, 1990.

Benson, Herbert, M.D., and Miriam Z. Klipper. *The Relaxation Response.* New York: Avon, 1990.

Burns, David D., M.D. *The Feeling Good Handbook.* New York: Plume, 1999.

Carnegie, Dale. *How to Stop Worrying and Start Living.* New York: Pocket Books, 1985.

Davis, Martha, Elizabeth Robbins Eshelman and Matthew McKay. *Relaxation & Stress Reduction Workbook.* Oakland, Calif.: New Harbinger Publications, 2000.

Goldberger, L., and S. Breznitz, eds. *Handbook of Stress: Theoretical & Clinical Aspects.* New York: Free Press, 1993.

Hand, I. and H. U. Wittchen, eds. *Panic & Phobias: Empirical Evidence of Theoretical Models and Long-Term Effects of Behavioral Treatments.* Berlin: Springer-Verlag, 1986.

_____, eds. *Treatments of Panic and Phobias: Modes of Application and Variables Affecting Outcome.* Berlin: Springer-Verlag, 1988.

Mavissakalian, M., and D. H. Barlow, eds. *Phobia: Psychological and Pharmacological Treatment.* New York: Guilford Press, 1981.

Meichenbaum, D. *Treating Post-Traumatic Stress Disorder.* New York: John Wiley, 1997.

Montgomery, Dr. Bob, and Dr. Laurel Morris. *Surviving: Coping with a Life Crisis.* Tucson, Ariz.: Fisher Books, 2000.

Nathan, P., and J. Gorman, eds. *A Guide to Treatments that Work.* New York: Oxford University Press, 1998.

O'Connor, Richard. *Undoing Depression: What Therapy Doesn't Teach You and Medication Can't Give You.* Boston: Little, Brown, 1997.

Parkinson, Frank. *Post-Trauma Stress: Restore Your Emotional Health.* Tucson, Ariz.: Fisher Books, 2000.

Pearsall, Paul, Ph.D. *A Healing Intimacy: The Power of Loving Connections.* New York: Crown Trade Paperbacks, 1995.

Potter-Efron, Ron, and Patricia S. Potter-Efron. *Letting Go of Anger: The 10 Most Common Anger Styles and What to Do About Them.* Oakland, Calif.: New Harbinger Publications, 1995.

Rachman, S., and J. D. Maser, eds. *Panic. Psychological Perspectives.* Hillsdale, N.J.: Erlbaum, 1988.

Schnarch, David. *Passionate Marriage: Love, Sex, and Intimacy in Emotionally Committed Relationships.* New York: Henry Holt, 1998.

Schnebly, Lee, M., ed. *Being Happy, Being Married.* Tucson, Ariz.: Fisher Books, 2001.

_____. *Nurturing Yourself and Others.* Tucson, Ariz.: Fisher Books, 2000.

Index